KNEE PAIN
AND DISABILITY

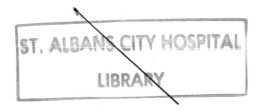

Other titles by Rene Cailliet from F.A. Davis Company:

Foot and Ankle Pain
Hand Pain and Impairment
Knee Pain and Disability
Low Back Pain
Scoliosis
The Shoulder in Hemiplegia
Shoulder Pain
Soft Tissue Pain and Disability
Head and Facial Pain Syndrome

KNEE PAIN AND DISABILITY
Edition 3

RENE CAILLIET, M.D.

Professor and Chairman Emeritus
Department of Physical Medicine and Rehabilitation
School of Medicine
University of Southern California
Los Angeles, California

Director
Rehabilitation Services
Santa Monica Hospital Medical Center
Santa Monica, California

Illustrations by R. Cailliet, M.D.

 F.A. DAVIS COMPANY • Philadelphia

F. A. Davis Company
1915 Arch Street
Philadelphia, PA 19103

Printed in the United States of America

Last digit indicates print number: 10 9 8 7 6 5 4 3 2

Note: As new scientific information becomes available through basic and clinical research, recommended treatments and drug therapies undergo changes. The author(s) and publisher have done everything possible to make this book accurate, up-to-date, and in accord with accepted standards at the time of publication. The authors, editors and publisher are not responsible for errors or omissions or for consequences from application of the book, and make no warranty, expressed or implied, in regard to the contents of the book. Any practice described in this book should be applied by the reader in accordance with professional standards of care used in regard to the unique circumstances that may apply in each situation. The reader is advised always to check product information (package inserts) for changes and new information regarding dose and contraindications before administering any drug. Caution is especially urged when using new or infrequently ordered drugs.

Library of Congress Cataloging-in-Publication Data

Cailliet, Rene.
    Knee pain and disability / Rene Cailliet ; illustrations by Rene Cailliet. —Ed. 3.
      p. cm.
    Includes bibliographical references and index.
    ISBN 0-8036-1622-8 (softbound : alk. paper) :
    1. Knee—Wounds and injuries. 2. Knee—Abnormalities.
    3. Knee—Diseases. 4. Pain. I. Title.
    [DNLM: 1. Knee. 2. Knee Injuries. WE 870 C134k]
    RD561.C34 1991
    617.5'82—dc20
    DNLM/DLC
    for Library of Congress   91-28232
                                              CIP

Preface to
Third Edition

The human knee has for centuries been exposed to numerous traumata, stresses, injuries, and diseases; but it appears that the recent generation has compounded the problem. Physical fitness programs intended for improving general health and cardiovascular conditioning have resulted in unacceptable knee problems. Competitive athletic activities have increased and simultaneously multiplied knee injuries. Vehicular accidents add their toll upon the knee, and with the increase in the aged population there are more people with degenerative knee changes.

Medical science and ancillary engineering sciences and ergonomic studies have afforded a better understanding of normal and abnormal knee function. Causes of injury can now be precisely reconstructed and the resultant tissues injured better understood.

By far the most illuminating in understanding, diagnosing, and properly treating the injured knee has been the advent of direct vision of internal knee structures through the arthroscope. CT Scanning and MRI studies now also reveal the soft tissues involved in injury in a noninvasive manner.

Proper immediate evaluation of the injured painful knee is now within the realm of the nonspecialized medical practitioner, chiropractor, athletic trainer, physical therapist, insurance carrier, and attorney facing these knee problems.

This totally rewritten text with numerous additional illustrations considers all aspects of the impaired painful knee in a concise, simple, practical, and constructive approach. The self-drawn illustrations by the author afford a visual aid to understanding what is otherwise a complicated mechanical articulation. The tissues responsible for pain and impairment are clearly described and their role in symptomatology made clearer. The clinical examinations that can precisely identify the injured tissue are precisely discussed and illustrated. Treatment protocols are no longer merely listed but their rationale is propounded and justified.

It is hoped that this book will enable the knee-injured patient to receive early appropriate recognition, undergo a meaningful examination, undergo significant tests, and receive appropriate medical care. The injured knee which can be the bane of the weekend to the professional athlete as well as the nonathlete should be pain-free for activities of daily living.

RENE CAILLIET M.D.

Preface to Second Edition

The human knee is subjected daily to numerous stresses, injuries, and diseases, and it places high in the percentage of patients disabled from musculoskeletal impairment in comparison with lumbrosacral pain, neck and shoulder pain, foot pain, and hand impairment. As stated in Chapter One, the knee is probably the most complicated joint in the human body.

Therefore, this book is offered in an effort to acquaint the student, intern, resident, family practitioner, and nonorthopedist with basic knee conditions they may see, often in the early phase of pain or disability. As in the previous CAILLIET PAIN SERIES, functional anatomy is stressed and illustrations are schematic for simplification and economy.

In order to maintain the small size of this book, neither exhaustive presentations of the subjects that are discussed in this book nor *all* knee conditions can be included. New forms of treatment constantly emerge and new concepts of disease and disability become clarified daily by continuing research and clinical experience. Only constant study can keep the practicing physician and therapist abreast of advancing scientific knowledge.

This new edition contains additional material relating to ligaments, cartilage, and gait mechanisms. New sections include ligamentous capsular injuries and patellofemoral arthralgia. Sections on nonsurgical treatment have been expanded upon. Thirty-one new illustrations have also been added.

It is hoped that this book will lead to earlier recognition of knee conditions, better evaluation, increased physiologic treatment, and earlier referral for more definitive and specialized treatment when so recognized.

RENE CAILLIET, M.D.

Contents

Illustrations

CHAPTER 1

Structural Anatomy

The knee joint is probably the most complicated joint in the human body. It is intricate because it comprises two structurally and functionally different yet interrelated joints: the tibiofemoral and patellofemoral joints. It is multidirectional in its movement, which is dictated by the planes of the opposing articular surfaces, the neuromuscular elements, and the ligamentous limiting actions. These structural and functional aspects of the knee joint must be thoroughly understood to obtain a meaningful evaluation and, when the knee is impaired, a meaningful therapy.

TIBIOFEMORAL ARTICULATION: OSSEOUS COMPONENTS

The tibiofemoral joint is formed by the distal end of the femur and the proximal surfaces of the tibia. The distal aspect of the femur has two surfaces (Fig. 1–1). Both are convex, asymmetrical, saddle-shaped condylar surfaces that are coated with cartilage. They are separated by a deep U-shaped notch, the intercondylar fossa. This fossa is deep and wide, equal in size to that of the average thumb.

The femur, viewed laterally, is flattened in its anterior surface and curved on its posterior aspect. The medial femoral condyle has a smaller transverse diameter (TM in Fig. 1–1) but a longer longitudinal length (LM in Fig. 1–1) than the lateral condyles. These femoral articular surfaces correspond to similar articular surfaces of the opposing tibial condyles. Cartilage covers a small part of the anterior curvature and the entire posterior surface of the inferior and posterior portion of the condyles. This cartilage has a thickness of 3 to 4 mm.

The tibial surface has two concavities. The articular concave surfaces are shallower than the convex femoral condyle, and these opposing articular

1

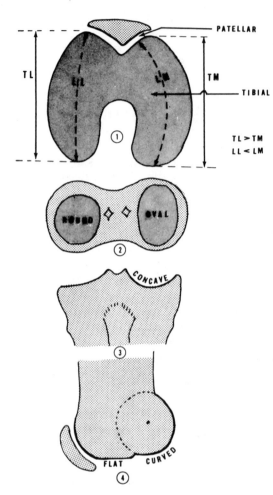

Figure 1-1. Knee joint surfaces. (*1*) Femoral condyle surfaces of the right knee. TL, Anteroposterior length of the lateral condyle; TM, Length of the medial condyle. The length of the medial condyle (LM) is greater than the length of the lateral condyle (LL) because of its curved surface. (*2*) Superior surface of the right tibia. The lateral articular surface is rounded and the medial articular surface is oval. (*3*) The medial tibial articular surface is deeper and more concave than is the lateral. (*4*) Side view of the femur showing the flat anterior surface and the curved posterior surface. The two articulations are illustrated in *1*. The patellar surface in which the patella articulates with the anterior femur and the tibial surface then glides upon the tibia.

surfaces are asymmetrical because of this difference in curvature. The medial tibial plateau faces inward and the lateral plateau faces outward; both face upward with two central bony spicules, the eminentia intercondylaris (Fig. 1–2), that extend into the fossa of the femur. These opposing articulating surfaces of the femoral condyles and the tibial plateau are incongruent or asymmetrical, and, thus, even though they are directly opposed and are in contact, they do not constitute a stable joint (Fig. 1–3).

MECHANICS OF JOINTS

Before specifically undertaking a discussion of the functional anatomy of knee joints, a discussion of the mechanics of joints per se merits considera-

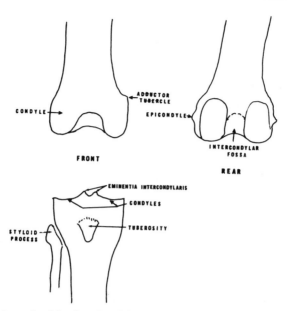

Figure 1–2. Superficial landmarks of the knee bones. (*Top*) femur; (*Bottom*) tibia.

tion. The understanding of joint mechanical function has benefitted by cooperation of the engineering profession and medicine. Physical treatment of joint dysfunction depends on a clear understanding of the mechanical function of any joint and its related tissues.

A typical synovial joint is formed by two opposing articular surfaces, each covered by cartilage, and enclosed within a capsule that contains synovial fluid, which is secreted as a lubricant by synovium. There are essentially two types of joint surfaces: ovoid and sellar (Fig. 1–4), with the ovoid surface being uniformly concave or convex.[1] The curvature of the opposing bone of the articulations is in turn either congruent or incongruent, depending on its arc or curvature and the structural relationship of the two surfaces.[2,3]

The ideal articulating surfaces of opposing bones comprising a joint are considered to be perfect curves that fit into each other with equal contact at each point along the articulating surfaces. Motion of this type of joint, a "true congruous joint," would occur around a fixed axis of rotation.

This definition of a true congruous joint is not accepted by engineering principles. Engineering studies of joints have shown that articular surfaces are variable rather than uniform. A true congruous joint would not permit lubrication of synovium whereas a degree of incongruity will move the lubricant to either side of the joint (Fig. 1–5).

A true congruous joint implies direct contact of the articular surfaces at every point around the curvature of the end surfaces. This contact creates a

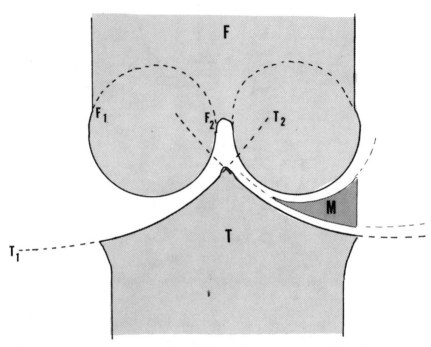

Figure 1–3. Incongruity of the femoral condyle curve to the tibial plateau curve (schematic). The convexity of the femoral condyles (F_1-F_2) is greater than the concavity of the tibial plateaus (T_1-T_2). This incongruity causes the interarticular joint space to be wider laterally than centrally. Normally, congruity is regained by the inclusion of a meniscus (M), which causes the articular surfaces to become parallel. In this schematic drawing only one meniscus is included, whereas normally there is one laterally and medially.

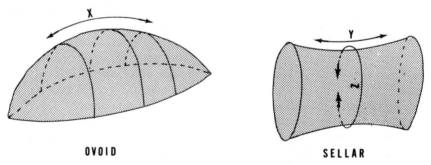

OVOID   SELLAR

Figure 1–4. Joint surfaces. There are two basic joint surfaces: ovoid and sellar. The ovoid is uniformly convex (X) at each point along the surface; the sellar surface is convex (Z) in one plane and concave (Y) in the perpendicular plane.

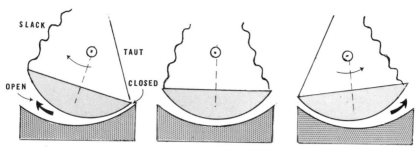

Figure 1–5. Asymmetrical joint surfaces. The asymmetrical joint surfaces of incongruous joints cause synovial fluid (*large arrow*) to flow toward the open articular area. The joint ligaments remain taut on the closing side and become slack on the opening side.

"close packed"[2] relationship and would "bind" the joint, that is, no lubrication would evolve (Fig. 1–6).

In an incongruous joint the articulating surfaces touch at varying sites and cover a small area. The remainder of the joint space is more separated (Fig. 1–6).

In the human body only the hip joint (femoral head into the acetabulum) approximates a congruous joint. This is the joint of greatest stability and yet limited motion. In this (congruous) joint the head of the femur is deeply "seated" within the acetabulum. The axis of rotation remains essentially in the center, and rotation (flexion, extension, abduction, adduction, and

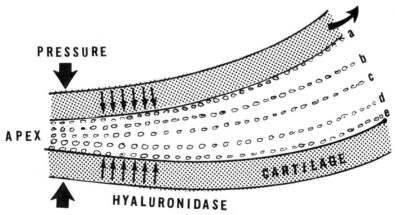

Figure 1–6. Hydrodynamic lubrication. Nonparallel joint surfaces form a wedge-shaped lubricating fluid, some of which stays at the apex. The lubricating fluid moves in layers—a, b, c, d, e—at the same speed as the articulating bone, but a layer (a–e) adheres to both articular surfaces. A shearing force between layers causes deformation of the fluid.

The lubricant is both adhesive and viscous, being coated by hyaluronic acid, which is created by the synovium and cartilage. Even without movement a layer(s) remains between the two opposing joint surfaces.

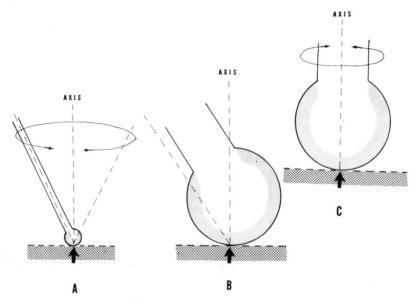

Figure 1–7. Joint motion: spin or rotation. True spin (*C*) is exemplified as in a spinning top about one point. If there is an angular change of the axis perpendicular (*A*) to the surface during spinning, a spin–rotation occurs (*B*).

internal-external rotation) evolves around this "fixed" axis centrum. Admittedly a congruous joint, true congruity is not possible, and thus the hip joint has a slight but definite incongruity.

    Motion of an incongruous joint is that of "spin" rather than roll or rotate (Fig. 1–7). This spin of the articulating joint surfaces combined with rotation,

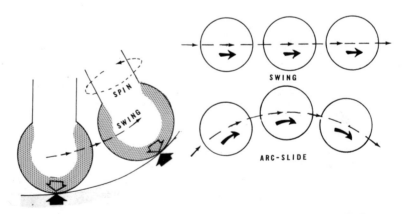

Figure 1–8. Joint motion. A joint sliding in one plane is termed "swing." This motion has no rotation or spin. If there is simultaneous spin, the motion is termed "arc slide."

which is what most joints do, especially the knee, results in an "arc-slide" (Fig. 1–8).

The capsule of a congruous joint is limited and shortens with rotation. The portion of the capsule that becomes extended on joint sliding or rolling may thicken and act to restrict motion in that direction. This thickened portion of the capsule veritably becomes a ligament (Fig. 1–9) and is evident in a standard joint but is not present in the knee joint (Fig. 1–10).

In a typical incongruous joint there is no deep seating of the joint surfaces. Thus, the muscles and ligaments must furnish support while simultaneously moving the convex surfaces on the concave surfaces. Both the ligaments and muscles are required for support and motion. In the knee, this does not occur. The ligaments supply the majority of the support, and the muscles supply the kinetic action.

Because the capsule attaches about the circumference of the concave socket and about the convex contour of the head and shaft, in a typical congruous joint, such as the femur, the capsule is the same length throughout and shortens symmetrically with motion. In an incongruous joint, the capsule is longer on one aspect and shorter in the other because the points of attachment differ as the head rotates. These capsular reactions are shown in Figure 1–11, which depicts gliding rotational motion in incongruous joints.

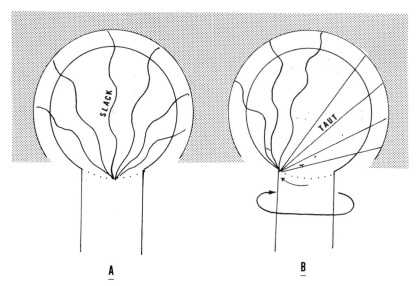

Figure 1–9. Capsular restriction of rotation. (A) The neutral position of a joint with the capsule is generally slack. With rotation of the bone (B), the capsule becomes taut and limits motion. The limiting capsular fibers may be enlarged enough to function as a ligament.

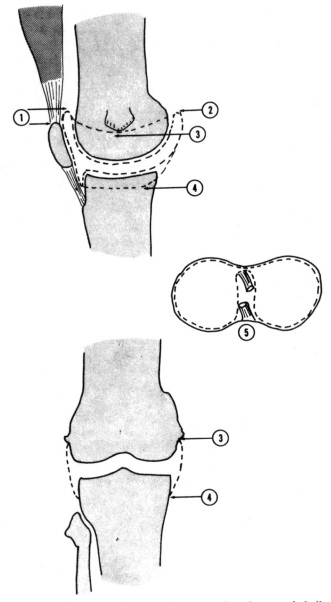

Figure 1–10. Synovial capsule. The knee joint capsule is large and shallow and can hold up to 40 ml of air without tension. (*1*) Anteriorly, it ascends to two finger breadths above the patella. (*2*) Posteriorly, it ascends to the origin of the gastrocnemius muscle. (*3*) Laterally, it attaches to the femur at the junction of the condylar cartilage at the epicondylar level. (*4*) Inferiorly, it attaches upon the tibia a quarter inch below the articular margin at the attachment of the collateral ligament. (*5*) The cruciate ligaments invaginate the capsule; thus they are *extracapsular*.

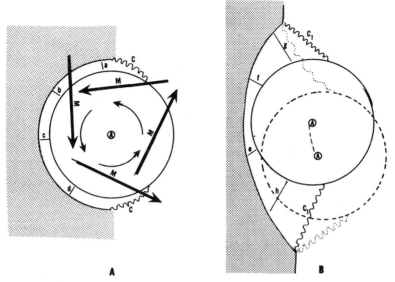

Figure 1-11. Congruous–incongruous joints. (*A*) In a congruous joint the concave and convex surfaces are symmetrical. The articular surfaces are equidistant from each other at all points along their circumference (a = b = c = d, etc.). In rotation, movement occurs about a fixed axis (A). Muscular action (M) is that of symmetrical movement about this fixed axis and is needed for motion, not stability. The depth of the concave surface gives the joint stability. The capsule (C) has symmetrical elongation. (*B*) Incongruous joints have asymmetrical articulatory surfaces. The concave surface is elongated and the convex more circular. This discrepancy makes the surface between the surfaces differ at various points along the circumference (g>f, e<h). As the joint moves, the axis of rotation (A) shifts and the joint glides rather than rolls. The muscles (M) move the joint and simultaneously stabilize it. The capsule (C) varies in its length. This is an example of an incongruous joint motion.

MENISCI

The tibiofemoral joint is incongruous and is thus mechanically relatively unstable. Congruity is achieved by the insertion of menisci into the joint between the femoral condyles and the tibial plateau (refer to Fig. 1–3).

Menisci are curved, wedge-shaped,[4] fibrocartilaginous pieces of tissue located on the periphery of the tibiofemoral joint, which are connected to each other and to the joint capsule. Their mechanical function is to assist in the distribution of pressure between the femur and the tibia in weight bearing and to balance the intra-articular pressure of muscular action. By creating a more congruous joint, they also assist in joint lubrication (refer to Fig. 1–5).

The medial meniscus is approximately 10 mm wide with its posterior horn wider than the middle portion (Fig. 1–12). The medial meniscus has a

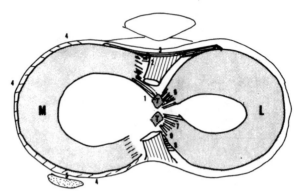

Figure 1–12. Attachments of the menisci. Right tibial plateau viewed from above. (*1*) Fibrous attachment of the medial meniscus (M) to outer ridge of the tibial tubercle (T). (*2*) Connection to the anterior cruciate ligament and (*3*) to the anterior horn of the lateral meniscus (L) via the ligamentous transversus. (*4*) The medial meniscus is attached around its entire periphery to the capsule and (*5*) posteriorly to the semimembranosus muscle tendon. The lateral meniscus has both its (*6*) anterior and (*7*) posterior horns attached to the eminentia intercondylaris (T) by a fibrous connection (*8*) to the posterior cruciate ligament. (*9*) A fibrous band attaches superiorly into the fossa intercondylaris of the femur.

wider curve than the lateral meniscus. Its anterior horn connects to the anterior ridge of the tibia by fibrous ligamentous tissue and to the ventral intercondylar spine. It often connects with the anterior cruciate ligament. By way of the ligamentous transversus, it connects to the anterior horn of the lateral meniscus. It is firmly connected around its periphery to the joint capsule and to the deep portion of the medial collateral ligament. Posteriorly, the medial meniscus connects to a fibrous thickening of the capsule and is also connected to the tendinous portion of the semimembranosus muscle (the posterior muscles of the thigh, i.e., the hamstrings).

The lateral meniscus has a width of 12 to 13 mm. Its curvature is greater than that of the medial meniscus, causing it to resemble a closed ring. In contrast, the medial meniscus is more C-shaped. Both the anterior and posterior horns of the lateral meniscus insert directly into the eminentia intercondylaris and by a fibrous connection to the posterior cruciate ligament (the ligamentous menisci fibularis). Most of the posterior horn inserts into the fossa intercondylaris femoris via a strong fasciculus that proceeds upward and medially. This fasciculus is known as the ligament of Wrisberg, which frequently blends with the posterior cruciate ligament.

The lateral meniscus has very loose connections to the lateral capsule. At its posterior horn, the popliteus tendon sheath is interposed between the lateral meniscus and the capsule. A synovial pouch (recessus inferior) exists between the meniscus and the capsule. Its outer wall forms a compartment (sheath) that contains the popliteus tendon. The lateral meniscus has great mobility essentially around the fulcrum attachments to the tibial spines with little or no lateral capsular connection.

BLOOD SUPPLY TO THE TIBIOFEMORAL JOINT STRUCTURES

There are five branches of the popliteal artery that supply vasculature to the knee joint. The femoral artery originates from the iliac artery in the femoral triangle of the groin and descends anteriorly, branching into the profundus femoris artery (Fig. 1–13), which branches further into four perforating arteries.[4]

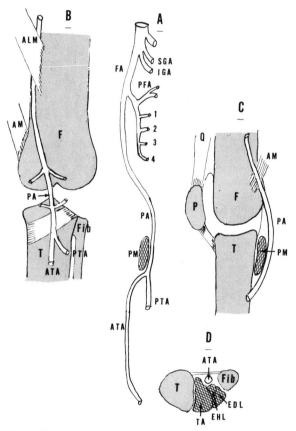

Figure 1–13. Femoral Artery. (A) Schematic of the femoral artery throughout the entire leg. (B) Posterior view of the knee region. (C) Lateral view of the knee region. (D) Superior view of the anterior compartment at mid-leg region. The entire arterial system is discussed in the text. F, femur; T, tibia; Fib, fibula; P, patella; ALM, adductor longus muscle; AM, adductor magnus (muscle); PA, popliteal artery; ATA, anterior tibial artery; PTA, posterior tibial artery; SGA, superior gluteal artery; IGA, inferior gluteal artery; PFA, profundus femoris artery; PM, popliteus muscle; TA, tibialis anterior (muscle); EHL, extensor hallucis longus (muscle); EDL, extensor digitorum longus (muscle); and Q, quadriceps (muscle).

The femoral artery descends over the adductor longus where it is posterior to the femur and proximal to the attachment of the adductus magnus muscle. The femoral artery becomes the popliteal artery at this point and proceeds between the femoral condyles.

As the popliteal artery approaches the popliteal space, it sends off two superior genicular arteries (Fig. 1–14), a central (middle) genicular artery, and, below the knee joint, two inferior genicular arteries. The superior genicular arteries curve around the femoral condyles proximal to the epicondyles and form a plexus in the suprapatellar area. The inferior genicular artery branches course around the margin of the tibial plateau, passing under the collateral ligaments. The middle genicular artery arises from the posterior portion of the popliteal artery, pierces the popliteal ligament, and sends three branches: the middle follows the anterior cruciate ligament and the medial and the lateral branches enter the perimeniscal connective tissue zone (Fig. 1–15).

The middle and inferior genicular branches supply the menisci, which are mostly avascular. Only the outer one third of the menisci has any significant blood supply. This vascularity plays a major part in recovery from any injury that may be sustained by the meniscus.

The superior genicular plexus is joined by the descending branch of the

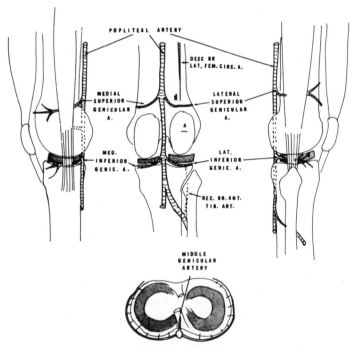

Figure 1–14. Blood supply of the knee joint. The popliteal artery has five branches in the area of the knee joint.

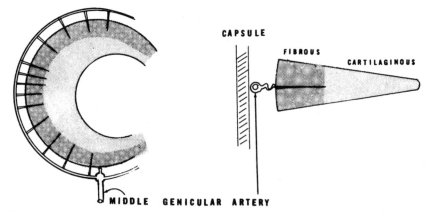

CAPSULE

FIBROUS

CARTILAGINOUS

MIDDLE GENICULAR ARTERY

Figure 1–15. Intrinsic circulation of the menisci. The middle genicular artery sends branches around the loose connective tissue of the perimeniscal zone under the capsule. Nonanastomatic small vessels, tortuous to permit movement, enter the fibrous zone (outer third) of the meniscus. They are more numerous in the central area of the meniscus. The inner third (cartilaginous zone) is avascular.

lateral femoral circumflex artery and the inferior genicular plexus is joined by the recurrent branch of the anterior tibial artery.

Over the popliteus muscle, the popliteal artery proceeds to divide into the anterior and posterior tibial arteries. The anterior tibial artery descends anteriorly within the compartment to join the anterior tibialis, the extensor hallucis longus, and the extensor digitorum longus muscles. In the foreleg, the anterior tibial artery lies on the septum that unites the tibia and the fibula, forming the posterior layer of the anterior compartment (Fig. 1–16).

LIGAMENTS

The incongruous bony configuration of the knee joint contributes little to the stability or integrity of the joint. The intrusion of the menisci improves the static stability[4] but has no effect on the kinetic component. The muscles impart motion to the joint but add little to the joint's stability. The capsule is redundant and essentially acts to contain the nutrient synovial fluid, but the capsule adds little to the joint's stability. Only the ligaments of the knee joint impart stability to the static and kinetic joint.

Ligaments are a type of connective tissue and have been extensively studied.[5] Ligaments are similar in structure and function to tendons except that the arrangement of the component collagen fibers in ligaments is more irregular than in tendons (Fig. 1–17). Ligaments also contain more elastin fibers within the collagen fibers. The anterior cruciate ligament, as an example, is made up of multiple fascicles of Type I collagen. The fibrils are

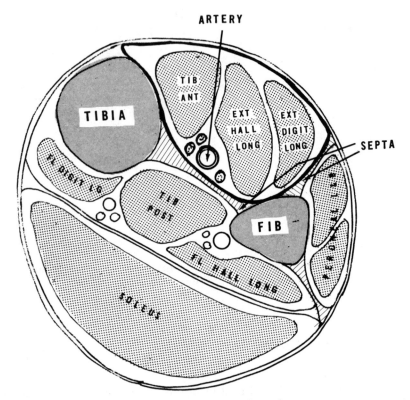

Figure 1–16. Anterior compartment of the lower leg. The anterior compartment is located within a fibrous sheath in the anterior portion of the lower leg. Posteriorly there is a firm fibrous septum between the tibia and the fibula. Within the compartment is located the tibial artery and veins and the anterior tibial, extensor hallucis longus, and the extensor digitorum longus muscles. Trauma to or compression of this compartment results in edema, which is firmly enclosed, and leads to drastic atrophy of the enclosed muscles and to compression nerve.

nonparallel, but the long axis of the fibers is oriented approximately longitudinally. Microscopically, as in all ligaments, the collagen fibers form a wavy, undulating pattern within a matrix that slowly straightens out on application of a load.

Tendons are similiar in gross structure. However, they have a greater cellular component, are metabolically more active, and contain fewer Type 3 collagen fibers and more cross linkage. Because of their composition, tendons can more readily be restored and are better able to recover from injury than ligaments; tendons are often employed for surgical replacement of damaged ligaments.[6]

The bony attachments of ligaments also play a part in normal use, trauma, and repair. Ligaments undergo a specific arrangement at their sites

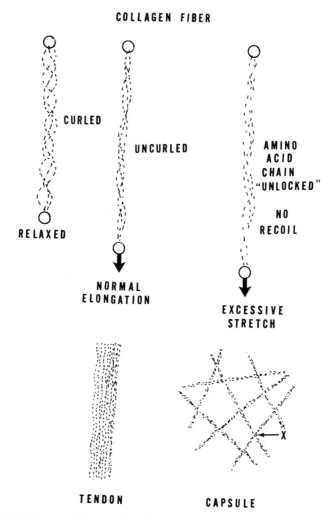

COLLAGEN FIBER

CURLED

UNCURLED

AMINO
ACID
CHAIN
"UNLOCKED"

NO
RECOIL

RELAXED

NORMAL
ELONGATION

EXCESSIVE
STRETCH

TENDON   CAPSULE

Figure 1–17. Collagen fiber. Each collagen fiber is a trihelical chain of amino acids bound together chemically. They uncurl to their physiological length, then recoil when the elongation force is released. If the collagen fiber is elongated past its physiological length, the amino acid chains become disrupted, and the fiber no longer returns to its resting length.

A tendon consists of parallel bands of collagen fibers. In a capsule, the collagen fibers crisscross and glide over each other at their intersection (X). The capsule depicted here elongates as far as each collagen fiber permits.

of attachment to bones. They merge from a region of greater parallelism (zone 1) into a fibrocartilaginous region (zone 2), then into a mineralized fibrocartilaginous region (zone 3), and then ultimately into bone (zone 4). These distal zones of attachment change the "stiffness" of the ligamentous attachment, which indicates why ligamentous failure is rare but bony avulsion is not.

The blood supply of ligaments, present in the embryo and neonatal life, involutes in adulthood, resulting in avascular ligaments. A ligament depends for its nutrition entirely on the vascularity of its synovial sheath, not on its bony attachment.

Ligaments of the knee receive nerve fibers from contiguous branches of the tibial nerve; the fibers serve as vasomotor fibers (sympathetic). However, recent studies[7,8] have alluded to the presence within ligaments of mechanoreceptors that have a role in proprioception.

Cruciate Ligaments

Of the knee ligaments, the collaterals and the cruciates, the cruciates have become recognized as being more important in assuring normal functioning. Damage to the cruciate ligaments contributes to significant impairment and disability.

Until recently, injury to this structure has often eluded recognition, evaluation, and proper treatment. Permanent impairment has resulted and the careers of many athletes have been terminated. More recent techniques of examination using arthroscopy, computerized tomography (CT), scanning, and magnetic resonance imaging (MRI) have determined the proper role of the cruciate ligaments in normal function and in pathology.

There are two cruciate ligaments: the anterior cruciate ligament (ACL) and the posterior cruciate ligament (PCL). The ACL is the more critical, and of the two most frequently involved in impairment or disability.

Anterior Cruciate Ligament. The ACL arises from the nonarticular aspect of the tibia and passes superiorly, laterally, and posteriorly to attach to the posterior portion of the intercondylar notch (Fig. 1–18). The ligament derives its label of "anterior" because it is located on the anterior surface of the tibia. The tibial attachment is long and firm, with some of its fibers arising from the medial and anterior aspect of the tibial spine (Fig. 1–19). Many fibers are attached to the anterior tip of the lateral meniscus and 20 percent reach posteriorly as far as the posterior tibial origin of the lateral meniscus.[9] The attachment to the femur is the posterior aspect of the medial surface of the lateral condyle. It is interesting that there are several reported cases of congenital absence of cruciate ligaments with apparent normal knee function,[10–12] which brings into question why traumatic impairment of the ACL causes such disability.

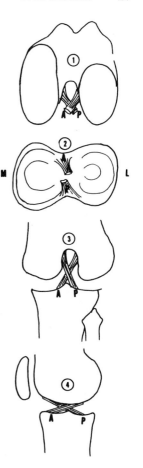

Figure 1–18. Cruciate ligaments. (*1*) Viewed from posterior aspect of right knee with knee bent. (*2*) Superior view of tibial plateau. (*3*) Posterior view of extended right knee. (*4*) Side view of knee.

A = Anterior ligaments
P = Posterior ligaments
M = Medial ligaments
L = Lateral ligaments

The ACL is composed of two bands: a small anteromedial band and a large bulky posterolateral band. These two bands travel parallel to each other and are attached along their lengths by a soft material that permits them to move differently.[13] This implies that different portions of the ligament tighten and loosen during movement of the knee and that there are parts of the ligament that remain taut constantly throughout this movement.

Vascular Supply.   Admittedly an avascular tissue, the ACL receives its blood supply from the inferior and middle genicular arteries (see Figs. 1–12 and 1–13). The synovium, and not the osseous ligamentous juncture, supplies the ligament's nutrition.[14,15]

The tensile strength of the anterior cruciate ligament has been equated to that of the collateral ligaments and is half that of the posterior cruciate ligament.[15,16]

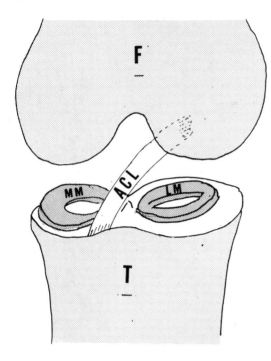

Figure 1–19. In a schematic depiction the cruciate ligament is shown angling from the inferior femoral (F) condyle to insert into the anterior aspect of the tibial (T) plateau. Its relationship to the menisci, medial MM and lateral LM, is depicted.

Function of the Anterior Cruciate Ligament. In the next chapter the functional anatomy of the total knee structure is discussed, but to relate structure to function (Fig. 1–20), the function of the ACL will be summarized.

The importance of the ACL remains controversial. There is a wide range of opinion; some believe it is relatively unimportant to the "essential stabilizer of the knee."[17] Most observers agree that the ACL:

1. Prevents anterior luxation. The ACL is responsible for 85 percent of the anterior displacement.[18]
2. Limits tibial rotation upon the femur.
3. Limits valgus and varus stress upon the knee.[19]

Only portions of the ACL function at any one time in preventing anterior luxation, but a portion of the ligament remains taut all the time. The anterior medial band (AMB) of the ligament provides resistance from 70° flexion to full flexion, and at 90° flexion the AMB is the major resistor. The posterior medial bands (PMBs) are taut in full extension and until 20° to 25° of flexion. Between 40° and 50° flexion neither bands are specifically taut, and in this range there is physiological anterior-posterior shear mobility.[20] Ligamentous failure has been calibrated to occur at 10 percent to 15 percent

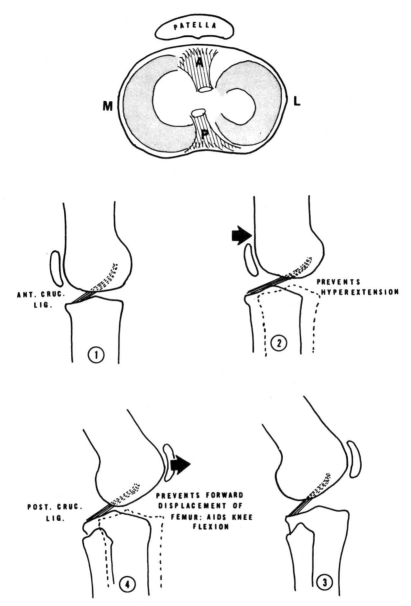

Figure 1–20. Function and restriction imposed upon cruciate ligaments. (*Top*) Superior view of the point of attachment and direction of the cruciates. Right knee medial aspect: (*1*) Direction of anterior cruciate and (*2*) method of preventing hyperextension of the knee. Right knee lateral aspect: (*3*) The posterior cruciate ligament and (*4*) manner in which it prevents forward displacement of the femur upon the tibia. By acting as a drag force it aids in normal knee flexion.

of ligamentous elongation.[21] Failure occurs more rapidly after any significant immobilization in which the ligaments are not being repeatedly stretched to their physiological limits.[22]

Rotation, especially internal rotation, of the tibia is limited by both bands of the ACL. Excessive rotation occurs after an injury to the ACL if there is concurrent injury to the lateral collateral ligament. In such a ligamentous injury, there may be injury to a meniscus. A pure single ligamentous instability is rarely encountered. As the center of rotation normally varies constantly during rotation this compounds the problem observed after injury.

The Posterior Cruciate Ligament

Throughout the medical orthopedic literature, the posterior cruciate ligament (PCL) remains obscure. As an isolated orthopedic injury it does not receive the attention in disabling orthopedic conditions as does the ACL (anterior cruciate ligament).

The PCL is intra-articular and extrasynovial with a crescentic insertion into the medial femoral condyle. Its thinner posterior portion fans out upon the posterior margin of the tibia. It is twice as strong as the anterior cruciate and acts reciprocally with the ACL.

The PCL functions basically as a knee stabilizer being most taut in midranges of knee motion. Some part of the PCL remains taut throughout all knee range of motion. It becomes the most taut in internal rotation of the tibia upon the femur in the weight-bearing leg, which is one of its major functions. It also resists hyperextension of the knee and assists in the medial stability of the knee.

In experimental division of the PCL and of the lateral ligaments, there occurs posterior tibial subluxation. Division of the PCL with simultaneous division of the medial ligaments there results in medial tibial condyle subluxation with posterior subluxation.

The strength of the PCL probably accounts for its infrequent involvement except in severe knee injuries that injure other knee structures. The PCL test is the reverse of the drawer sign depicted in the previous section on the ACL with the flexed knee permitting the tibia to move excessively posteriorly.

Capsular and Collateral Ligaments

The capsule of the knee joint is essentially a thin fibrous membrane that is "reinforced" into fascial ligamentous structures that stabilize the knee. These collateral ligaments stabilize the joint by guiding as well as restricting joint motion. They can be divided into medial and lateral portions (Fig. 1–21), each having specific characteristics.

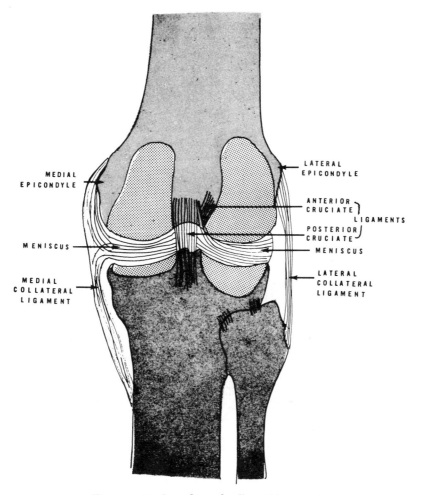

Figure 1–21. Capsular and collateral ligaments.

Medial Collateral Ligaments. Unlike the cruciate ligaments the medial collateral "ligament" is not a distinct ligament. This ligament consists of essentially three layers of fascialike tissues on the medial side of the knee. They attach superiorly to the femoral medial epicondyle and inferiorly to the tibia just below the level of the articular cartilage.

Layers 1 to 3 consist of deep fascia (crural), the superficial medial ligament, and the capsule and deep medial portion, respectively.[23] Layer 1 is a fascia immediately under the skin that extends anteriorly to enclose the patella and its tendon and posteriorly to enclose the popliteal fossa. The sartorius muscle inserts into the fascia but does not have its own tendon. The gracilis and semitendinosus muscles have distinct tendons that invaginate the fascia.

Layer 2 is the superficial medial ligament (Fig. 1–22). The fibers are parallel and vertical, but as they continue posteriorly, they tend to become more oblique where they merge with layer 3 and with the tendon sheath of the semimembranosus muscle. The anterior fibers of layer 2 merge, forming the patellofemoral ligament, which joins the patella to the femur.

The deep section of the medial collateral ligament essentially divides into three portions: the anterior, middle, and posterior ligaments (as shown

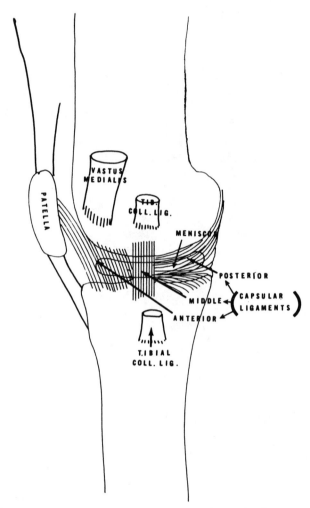

Figure 1–22. Medial (tibial) superficial collateral ligament. The three segments of the deep medial capsular ligament are shown: the parallel fibers of the anterior portion, the middle vertical, and the fanned indistinct posterior fibers. The superficial collateral ligament attaches just superior to the femoral medial epicondyle and to the tibia just below the articular cartilage and posterior to a point above the insertion of the semimembranous tendon.

in Fig. 1–20). The anterior portion of the fibers extends anteriorly into the extensor mechanism and has a loose connection with the anterior horn of the medial meniscus. These fibers are relaxed during knee extension but become taut during knee flexion (Fig. 1–23). They play a role in maintaining the alignment of the patella within the femoral condylar groove in knee actions.

The middle portion of layer 2 has been called the medial collateral ligament, the tibial collateral ligament, the superficial medial collateral ligament, the superficial medial ligament, or the internal collateral ligament. It is best termed "the parallel fibers of the superficial medial ligament"[24]

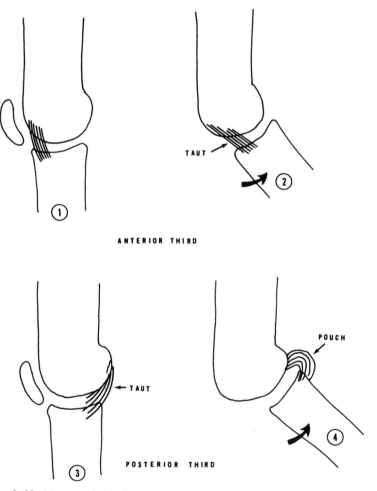

ANTERIOR THIRD

POSTERIOR THIRD

Figure 1–23. Motion of the deep medial ligaments during knee flexion. (*1*) The anterior fibers are slightly slack during knee extension and (*2*) taut during flexion. (*3* and *4*) The opposite action of the posterior fibers.

(Fig. 1–20). This portion of the medial ligament is roughly 11 cm long and 0.5 cm wide.

The middle portion of the medial ligament is in turn divided into two sections (Fig. 1–24): the superior meniscofemoral segment, which is thick and fixes the medial meniscus, and the inferior meniscotibial segment, which is loose and permits the tibia to move on the meniscus.

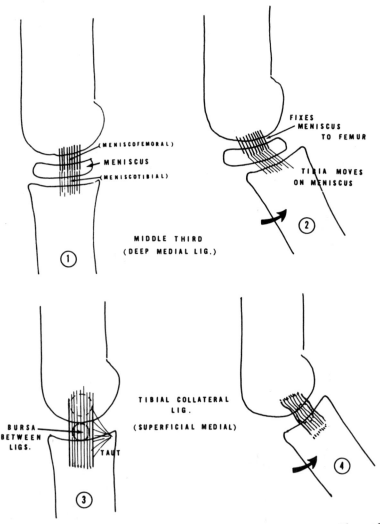

Figure 1–24. Deep medial and superficial collateral ligamentous action. The middle segment of the deep medial capsular ligament is divided into (1) a superior portion that fixes the medial meniscus to the femur during flexion and (2) an inferior portion that is slack and permits the meniscus to move. Joint spaces called meniscofemoral and meniscotibial are arbitrarily formed. (3 and 4) The relationship of a bursa to the superficial and deep medial ligaments is shown.

Layer 3 is the capsule. There has been controversy as to whether the capsule is a blend of deep retinacular tendons and synovial thin capsular tissues or is a separate entity. The latter alternative appears correct since the capsule and ligament are separable.[23]

Lateral Ligaments. The lateral compartment of the knee extends posteriorly from the lateral margin of the patellar tendon to the posterior cruciate ligament and is divided into three areas: the anterior, middle, and posterior.[25] Superiorly it attaches to the lateral epicondyle of the femur and inferiorly to the head of the fibula (Fig. 1–25).

The anterior area consists of the capsule, extending from the patellar tendon to the anterior margin of the iliotibial band and the lateral expansion of the quadriceps tendon. This portion of the lateral knee ligament is functionally more important to the patellofemoral mechanism than to knee stability.

The middle area of the lateral compartment is the iliotibial band, which covers the capsular ligament. This ligament, in turn, consists of a meniscotibial and a meniscofemoral portion. The iliotibial band connects to the lateral epicondyle of the femur, then to the lateral tubercle of the tibia. It is this posterior aspect of the iliotibial band that can actually be considered the lateral collateral ligament (Fig. 1–25). Being ahead of the axis of rotation of the femoral condyle (○ in Fig. 1–26), the lateral collateral ligament extends the knee and is a major knee support until 30° of flexion. It allows normal rotation when it is relaxed in flexion and becomes taut when it is in full rotation.

The posterior portion of the lateral compartment consists of inderdigitating fibers of the capsule and the fascial fibers emanating from the iliotibial band. These fibers are collectively termed the "arcuate ligamentous complex" and contain the tendon of the popliteus muscle (Fig. 1–25). The popliteus muscle has three tendinous origins and ultimately inserts via a muscular belly into the posterior proximal tibia. The three tendinous origins arise from the lateral femoral condyle, the posterior aspect of the fibula, and the posterior horn of the lateral meniscus. These tendinous origins form a Y-shaped ligament. The biceps tendon inserts into the fibular head, capsule, iliotibial band, and lateral collateral ligament. The posterior capsular compartment tightens when the knee extends and relaxes on flexion.

The arcuate ligament lies over the popliteal fascia and is firmly attached to it. The posterior fossa of the knee is bounded superiorly by the semimembranosus, semitendinosus, and the biceps tendon and inferiorly by the two heads of the gastrocnemius muscle. The roof of the fossa is the popliteal fascia. The peroneal nerve passes the neck of the fibula behind the biceps tendon. The fossa contains the popliteal artery, vein, and nerve. In the upper portion of the fossa, the popliteal nerve divides into the tibial and peroneal branches, which pass over the lateral head of the gastrocnemius muscle and under the fascia.

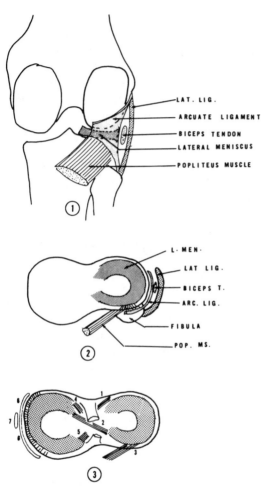

LAT. LIG.
ARCUATE LIGAMENT
BICEPS TENDON
LATERAL MENISCUS
POPLITEUS MUSCLE

L·MEN·
LAT LIG.
BICEPS T.
ARC. LIG.
FIBULA
POP. MS.

Figure 1–25. Lateral ligaments of knee. (*1*) The deep part of the lateral ligament attaches from the femoral epicondyle to the styloid process and tibial border of the fibular head. The posterior border lying across the popliteus muscle forms the arcuate ligament. The arcuate ligament attaches firmly to the posterior horn of the lateral ligament. Between the lateral ligament attachment and the arcuate ligament passes the tendon of the biceps femoris muscle. (*2*) The popliteus muscle emerges beneath the arcuate ligament to insert medioposteriorly on the tibia. The muscle originates partly from the arcuate ligament margin and from the posterior aspect of the meniscus. When the knee flexes, this muscle probably pulls the meniscus and simultaneously externally rotates itself, thus protecting the meniscus. (*3*) Attachment of menisci. The lateral menisci are attached at both horns to the tibia (1–2) with 2 crossing over from the posterior horn of the lateral meniscus to the anterior horn of the medial meniscus and the femoral attachment of the anterior cruciate ligament. There are fibrous bands (1–4) that connect anterior horns of both menisci to the femoral attachments of the anterior cruciate. The medial meniscus is attached by its anterior and posterior horns with fibrous bands 4–5, and along the entire circumference of the capsule (6) and the superficial medial ligament (7).

MUSCLES OF THE KNEE JOINT

The knee is powerfully motored and stabilized by numerous muscles that cross the joint anteriorly, posteriorly, and on either side. They are functionally designated as the anterior *extensor*, posterior *flexor*, medial *adductor*, and lateral *abductor* groups. The abductors and the adductors are rotators and stabilizers.

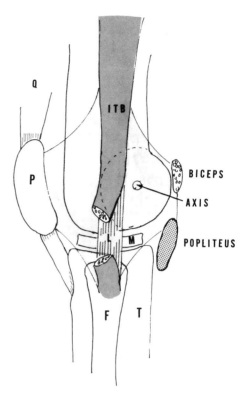

Figure 1–26. Lateral collateral ligamentous structures. The following are components of the lateral ligamentous compartment of the knee: P = patella; T = tibia; F = fibula; Q = quadriceps; ITB = iliotibial band; L = lateral collateral ligament; and M = meniscus (lateral). The axis is that of rotation of the femoral condyles in knee flexion. The iliotibial band is divided and pulled away to expose the lateral ligament.

Anterior Muscles

The major muscle of the extensor group is the quadriceps femoris, which comprises the rectus femoris and three vasti muscles termed the medialis, lateralis, and intermedius (Fig. 1–27) muscles. The rectus femoris muscle originates as a tendon from the inferior iliac spine of the pelvis, which is immediately superficial to the iliac origin of the iliofemoral ligament of the hip joint (Fig. 1–28). By crossing the hip joint, the rectus femoris exerts flexor forces. The vasti all originate from the anterior surface of the femur. The extensor group converges on a ligament that attaches to the tibial tuberosity of the tibia. At its termination, the extensor group has incorporated into its tendon a sesamoid bone, the patella (Fig. 1–29), forming the *other* joint of the knee, the patellofemoral knee joint.

Quadriceps Function. Since the quadriceps muscles are so important in normal kinetics of the knee joint as well as contributing to impairment and dysfunction of the knee, quadriceps function merits special study. Patients who sustain a knee injury commonly demonstrate early atrophy of the vastus medialis segment of the quadriceps and frequently lack strength and full extension of the knee. These findings have led to speculation as to which

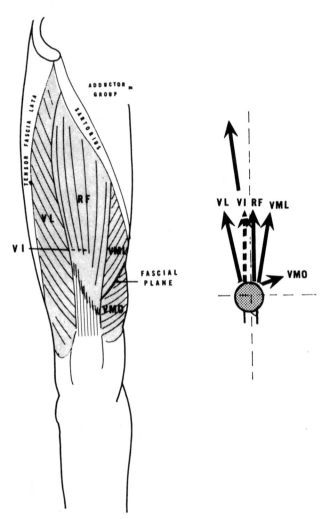

Figure 1–27. Quadriceps femoris: function of quadriceps mechanism. Each long component of the quadriceps group (RF, rectus femoris; VL, vastus lateralis; VI, vastus intermedius; VM, vastus medialis) can extend the knee fully. The vastus medialis oblique fibers (VMO) cannot extend the knee but apparently pull the patella medially (right) and keep it centered against lateral pull of the quadriceps (*arrows*). All long components pull equally throughout extension range with VMO exerting twice the force of contraction. The mechanics of the joint determine weakness (less efficiency) in the last 15° to 20°.

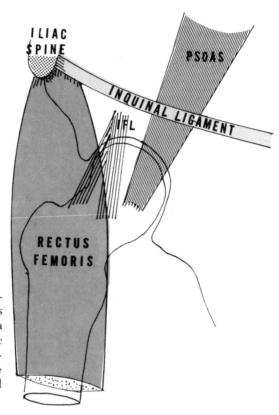

Figure 1–28. Origin of the rectus femoris muscle. The rectus femoris muscle originates as a tendon from the inferior iliac spine and the origin of the inquinal ligament. It overlays the iliofemoral ligament (IFL) and descends across the hip joint.

aspect of the quadriceps muscle group is vital to full extension throughout its range of motion. It has also led to many pathomechanical investigations of the patellar function in knee extension and flexion, which is considered in the chapter on gait.

As shown in Fig. 1–26, the alignment of the fibers of the vastus medialis longus and the longitudinal axis of the femur differ by approximately 15°, whereas the oblique fibers of the vastus medialis differ by 50° to 55°, being almost horizontal. For several decades we believed that the vastus medialis muscle contracted in the last several degrees of extension; recent evidence indicates otherwise. Electromyographic studies[25,26] have revealed contraction of all parts of the quadriceps groups throughout the range of 0° to 90° of flexion. This is also true for patients who have had recent surgery and who have chronic quadriceps deficit.[27]

The knee can be extended by any of the individual components of the quadriceps: the vastus lateralis, vastus intermedius, vastus medialis longus, and rectus femoris. The knee cannot be extended merely by the oblique fibers of the vastus medialis. Interestingly, 60 percent more force is required for the last 15° of extension than is required up to that degree of extension. If the oblique fibers contract to center the patella in its femoral groove, then 13 percent less force is needed.[28] It would appear from this that the oblique fibers function primarily in seating the patella. There also appears to be no significant difference in the force exerted by the various fibers of the quadriceps in knee extension. The apparent difference is dictated by the mechanical advantage of the intrusion of the patella in the extensor

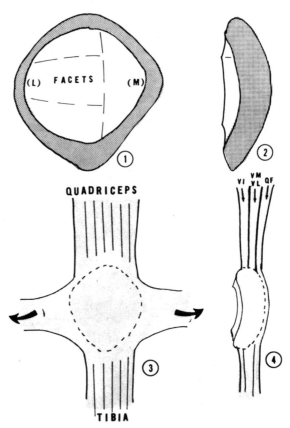

Figure 1–29. Patella. (*1*) Ventral view showing the articular surfaces divided into three medial facets and a lateral facet that articulate with the femur. The lateral aspect is wider than the medial. The rough bone presents the surface upon which the patellar extensor mechanism attaches. (*2*) Lateral view of the patella. (*3*) The quadriceps attaches to the patella. Laterally and medially (*arrows*), fibers extend to attach to the femoral condyles and the capsulomeniscal tissues. (*4*) The three layers of the tendinous insertion. The quadriceps (QR) covers the anterior aspect of the patella. The vasti medialis and lateralis (VM and VL) attach to the middle (superior and lateral) aspects of the patella and the vastus intermedius (VI) to the posterior (superior) margin.

mechanism and the effort of the quadriceps (oblique fibers) to maintain the patellar alignment.

Patellofemoral Joint. The patella is a sesamoid bone contained within the quadriceps tendon (Fig. 1–29) that participates in the mechanical activity of the quadriceps (Fig. 1–30). It comprises the knee joint as well as the tibiofemoral joint, but the patella influences the function of this latter joint (Fig. 1–31). The quadriceps femoris tendon is formed of three lamina: the superficial layer of the rectus, the middle layer from tendons of the vastus lateralis and medialis, and a deep layer from the vastus intermedius. Some of these tendon fibers pass anteriorly to the patella, some attach to the superior margin, and some to the lateral margins. Fibers from both the medial and the lateral aspects fan out to attach to the femoral condyles, while others pass to the capsular collateral ligaments (see Fig. 1–29).

The inner surface of the patella is covered with cartilage and glides on the cartilage of the femoral condylar notch. Here again we are dealing with an incongruous joint relationship. The asymmetric infrapatellar surfaces vary in their contact with the femoral condyles as the knee flexes and extends.

The facets of the patella make contact with the femoral condyles

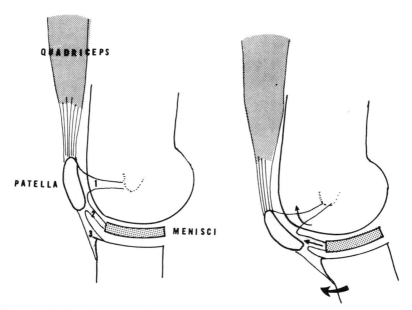

Figure 1–30. Quadriceps mechanism. The quadriceps extends over the anterior knee joint with three ligamentous extensions: (1) the epicondylopatellar portion attaches to the epicondyle eminence of the femur and guides rotation of the patella; (2) the meniscopatellar attaches to and pulls the meniscus forward during knee extension; and (3) the infrapatellar tendon, which attaches to the tibial tubercle and extends the tibia upon the femur.

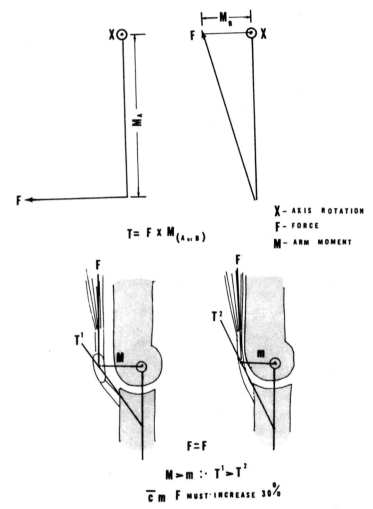

Figure 1–31. Mechanical function of the patella. (*Top*) Parallelograms of forces. When force is applied perpendicular to arm to rotate around axis (X), torque (T) equals force (F) times length of arm (M_A). With force applied oblique to arm, the moment becomes the distance from the force to the axis; thus, $T = F \times M_B$. (*Bottom*) In the knee, the patella increases the arm moment from m to M and thus torque T^1 is greater than T^2 with similar force (F). If the patella is not present, it has been calculated that a 30 percent increase in quadriceps strength is necessary to create equal torque. These forces are computed to knee rotation but disregard translation (gliding).

differently at various degrees of flexion.[29] At 20° of flexion the contact is a small area of the upper pole of the patella (Fig. 1–32). By 45° of flexion the middle portion of the lateral facets make contact, and at 90° of flexion the contact is entirely on the inferior lateral facet. At 45° of flexion the patella is the only tissue separating the quadriceps from the femoral condyles, and

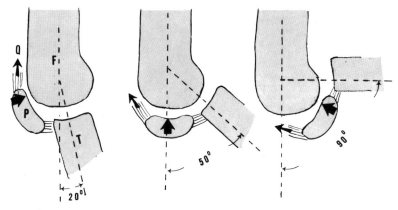

Figure 1–32. Patellar contacts upon knee flexion. With the knee flexed to 20°, the contact (*arrow*) with the femoral (F) condyles is on the upper portion of the patella (P). With 50° of flexion, the pressure is midpoint on the patella, and with 90° of flexion, the contact is upon the lower third of the patella. Q depicts the quadriceps, which exerts tension upward upon the tibia (T).

thus, only a small point of contact of the patella sustains all the weight of the body during knee flexion.

The odd facet (medial) on the medial aspect of the ridge separating the facets (Fig. 1–27) does not make contact with the femoral condyles until 135° of flexion. The medial facet makes contact with the medial femoral after 135° of flexion when the patella has undergone rotation and is in the intercondylar notch condyle.

The nerve supply of the quadriceps is the femoral nerve, which is formed by the anterior primary division of the L_{2-4} nerve roots (Fig. 1–33). Besides being motor to the quadriceps, it furnishes a major cutaneous branch to the medial side of the leg and foot. Its major function activates the knee jerk. The sensory division of the femoral nerve showing the dermatomes of C2, C3, and C4 are shown in Figure 1–34. A typical nerve root showing the entry of the sensory nerve to the spinal cord via its dorsal root ganglion is shown in Figure 1–35.

The sartorius muscle (Fig. 1–36), in addition to the quadriceps group, is part of the anterior thigh muscle group. This ribbonlike muscle spirals across the thigh from its origin at the anterior superior spine to the anterosuperior medial portion of the tibia below the anterior tuberosity. When this muscle is contracted, the individual assumes the position of a seated tailor (hence the name sartorius): the hip flexed, abducted and laterally rotated with the knee flexed and medially rotated. In its proximal region the sartorius (along with the adductor longus) forms the lateral margin of the femoral triangle.

The tensor fascia lata (Fig. 1–36) originates from the lateral aspect of the pelvis and descends along the lateral thigh region across the knee. This

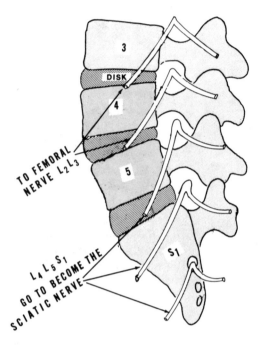

Figure 1–33. Sciatic nerve roots. The fourth and fifth lumbar nerves and the sacral nerve form the sciatic nerve. This nerve goes down the back of the leg to the foot and toes. The second and third lumbar nerves do *not* go into the sciatic nerve. They merge to form the femoral nerve, which goes down the *front* of the thigh to the thigh muscles. (Modified from Cailliet, R: Understand Your Backache. FA Davis, Philadelphia, 1984, p 81.)

occurs just ahead of the axis of rotation (small ○ in Fig. 1–36) where the tensor fascia lata forms a portion of the lateral collateral ligament, which was previously described in this chapter. Its being ahead of the knee rotation axis implies that it acts to extend the knee in the standing position to stabilize it laterally.

Posterior Thigh Muscles

The posterior thigh and lower leg muscles that cross the knee both flex and rotate the leg on the femur. The posterior thigh muscles are best divided into the medial and lateral groups (Fig. 1–37), which are termed the "hamstring muscles." The medial group contains the semimembranosus and semitendinosus muscles, which, when flexed internally, rotate the lower leg on the femur. The biceps femoris is the main lateral muscle of the hamstring group, and when the knee is flexed it internally rotates the lower leg on the femur (Fig. 1–38).

The semimembranosus muscle originates from the ischial tuberosity of the pelvis (see Fig. 1–36), blending with the origin of the long head of the biceps femoris muscle. The semimembranosus muscle descends along the medial aspect of the femur, crosses the knee joint, and inserts by a thick divided tendon containing four branches (Fig. 1–39). The major branch

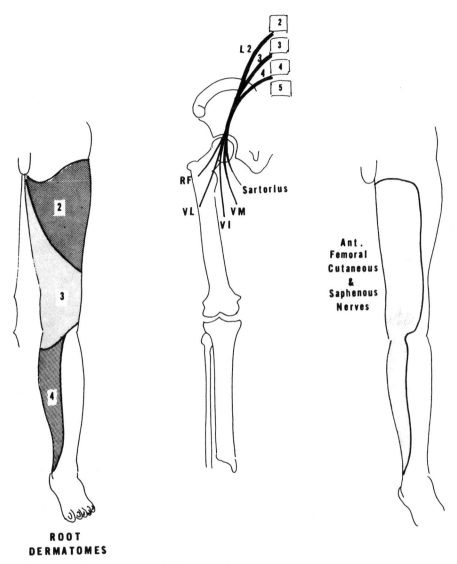

ROOT DERMATOMES

Figure 1–34. Distribution of the femoral nerve: its root formation. (*Left*) Root dermatomes of the leg and thigh. (*Center*) Formation of the nerve with anterior primary divisions of L_2, L_3, and L_4. (*Right*) Cutaneous sensory distribution of the lower extremity.

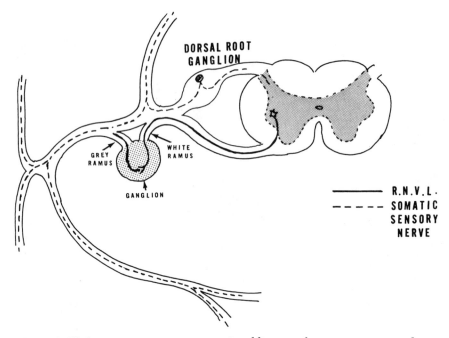

Figure 1–35. Somatic sensory nerve root. In addition to the recurrent nerve of von Luschka (R.N.V.L.) which innervates the low back, sensory transmission of nociceptive stimuli of the knee ascend via the somatic sensory nerve (dotted line) through the dorsal root ganglion. Sensory impulses then enter the dorsal gray matter of the cord.

inserts into the medial surface of the tibia beneath the medial ligament of the knee. This tendon sends fibers into the popliteus and the medial meniscus. By means of these attachments, the semimembranosus muscle flexes the knee, internally rotates the flexed leg, and pulls the medial meniscus backward to accompany the tibia during knee flexion.

The semitendinosus muscle also originates from the ischial tuberosity and inserts into the medial surface of the tibia in a vertical line immediately posterior to the sites of attachment of the sartorius and gracilis muscles. These three muscles form a conjoined tendon called the "pes anserinus" (Fig. 1–40). Under this tendon is a bursa that is a frequent site of inflammation and pain tenderness.[30]

The lateral knee flexor of the hamstring group is the biceps femoris muscle. The long head originates from the ischial tuberosity and descends across the posterior femur, merging along the way with the short head of the biceps that originates from the linea aspera of the femur. All the hamstring muscles, except the short head of the biceps, cross two joints in their course.

The long head of the biceps muscle forms a broad flat tendon 7 to 10 cm above the level of the knee joint, where it is joined by the fleshy tendon of

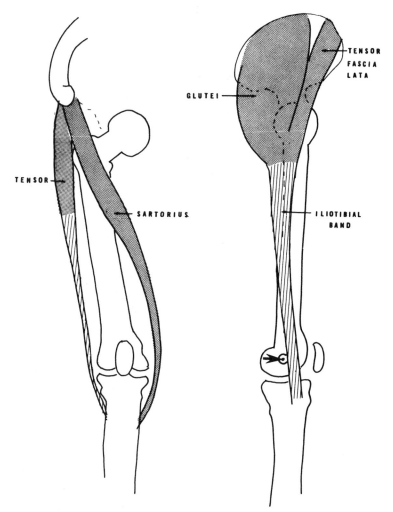

Figure 1–36. Sartorius muscle: tensor fascia lata. The sartorius muscle is a weak flexor of the knee and hip. The tensor fascia lata, which acts upon the knee, is considered to be a knee extensor but its primary function is abduction and stabilization of the hip.

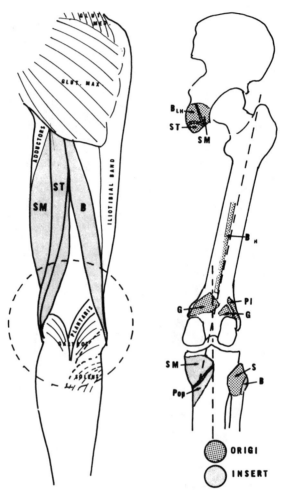

Figure 1–37. Posterior thigh muscles: flexors. (*Left*) The semimembranosus (SM), semitendinosus (ST), and the biceps femoris (B). The other muscles are labeled. (*Right*) The origin and insertion of the posterior muscle groups.

B_{LH} = Biceps long head
B_{SH} = Biceps short head
B   = Biceps
S   = Sartorius
Pl   = Plantaris
Pop = Popliteus
G   = Heads of gastrocnemius

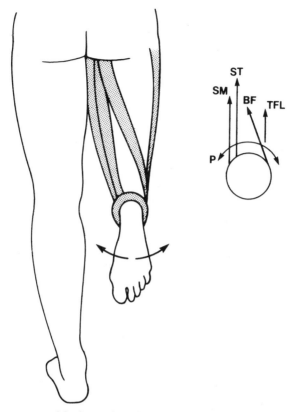

Figure 1–38. Rotators of the leg. When the knee is flexed the semimembranosus (SM) and the semitendinosus (ST) inwardly rotate the tibia. The biceps femoris (BF) and the tensor fascia lata (TFL) externally rotate the leg. The popliteus (P), originating laterally and inserting medially, internally rotates the leg upon the femur.

the deep head. It then splits into three tendinous inserts (Fig. 1–41): the superficial, middle, and deep inserts. The superficial layer in turn forms three expansions: the anterior, middle, and posterior expansions (Fig. 1–42). The anterior is thin, yet resilient, and fans out forward and downward into the lower leg. The middle expansion is also thin and divides to surround the lateral collateral ligament from which it is separated by bursae. The posterior expansion is connected to the collateral ligament and to the joint capsule by a firm fibrous band. The "deep layer" bifurcates into a fibular and tibial ligament and then attaches to the fibular head and the posterior aspect of the joint capsule. Both the superficial and deep layers send fibers anteriorly to attach to the infrapatellar ligament and help direct the motion of the patella.[27]

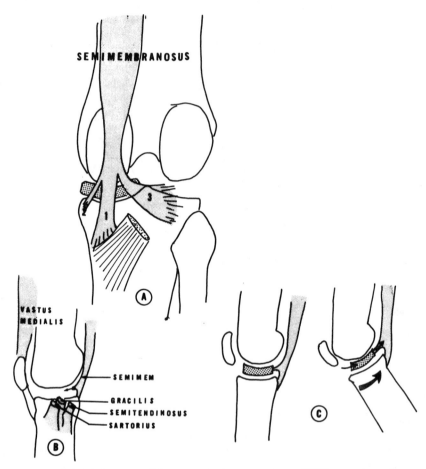

Figure 1–39. Medial aspect of the posterior knee structure. (A) The semimembranosus muscle has four tendinous inserts. The major insert (1) extends to attach on the posterior aspect of the tibia and sends fibers into the popliteus. In its path there is an exterior branch that attaches to the posterior aspect of the medial meniscus (2 and 3). These tendons complete the posterior popliteal fossa and tense the capsule. (B) The medial aspect of the knee with the insertion sites of the medial flexors. (C) The semimembranosus flexes the knee and simultaneously pulls the meniscus backward and rotates it with the tibia.

The biceps femoris muscle flexes the knee, and when the knee is flexed, the biceps femoris externally rotates the tibia upon the femur. As the knee flexes, the middle layer of its insertion, which surrounds the collateral ligament (see Fig. 1–42) causes this ligament to become slack. By its attachment of the deep layer to the capsule, this middle layer prevents impingement of the capsule between the tibia and femur as the knee flexes. This expansion is also attached to the iliotibial band (tensor facia lata) and aids

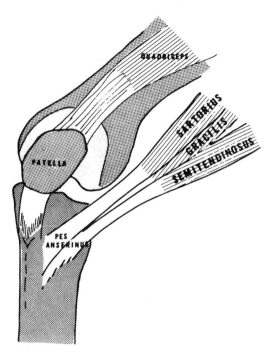

Figure 1–40. Pes anserinus. The medial insertion of the outer hamstring group forms a conjoined tendon of the semitendinosus with the sartorius and the gracilis muscles to form the pes anserinus. This tendon is separated from the underlying femoral condyle by a bursa.

in keeping it taut during the full range of knee flexion, especially between 10° to 30° of flexion.

Nerve Supply.   The flexor muscles receive their nerve supply from the sciatic nerve. The sciatic nerve divides into the tibial and common peroneal nerves above the knee joint just below the inferior margin of the long head of the biceps muscle. The tibial nerve supplies the semimembranosus, semitendinosus, and long head of the biceps. The common peroneal branch supplies the short head of the biceps.

Popliteus Muscle.   The popliteus muscle forms a part of the floor of the posterior knee fossa and arises from the lateral epicondyle of the femur and runs posteromedially to attach by numerous fleshy bands into the posterior aspect of the tibia. Some of the fibers attach to the lateral meniscus.[31] The function of the popliteus muscle is to rotate the tibia internally. It is a very weak knee flexor.

Posterior Calf Muscles

The gastrocnemius muscle arises from two flattened, largely tendinous heads: the medial and lateral heads. The lateral head arises from the epicondyle of the femur just above the origin of the popliteus and the attachment of the fibular collateral ligament. The medial head arises from

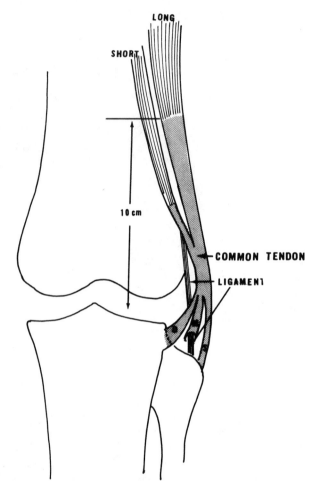

Figure 1–41. Biceps femoris tendon. The long head remains fleshy until about 10 cm above the knee joint, where it becomes a flat tendon. The short head remains fleshy until the fibular head. The common tendon then splits into three layers: superficial (S), middle (M), and deep (D).

above the medial condyle from the popliteal surface. The heads quickly unite, descend the lower leg, and join the soleus muscle, which originates from the tibia and fibula. At midleg they terminate into the achilles tendon, which attaches to the calcaneus.

There is a constant bursa present between the tendon of the semimembranosus muscle and the medial head of the gastrocnemius, which occasionally communicates with the capsule of the knee joint. As a sequela of a sprain, which causes effusion in the knee joint, fluid may pass into the bursa behind

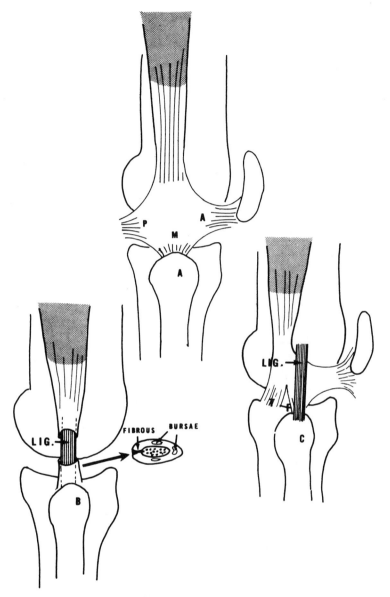

Figure 1–42. Layers of the common biceps tendon. (*A*) Superficial layer. The tendon divides into three expansions: anterior (A), which fans out to blend with the anterior crural fascia; middle (M), which extends to the collateral ligament at the fibular head; posterior (P), which blends with the fascia of the calf and lateral leg muscles. (*B*) Middle layer. This is a thin layer that splits to envelop the lateral collateral ligament. The insert depicts the relationship of the bursae and the posterior fibrous attachment to the ligament. (*C*) Deep layer. This layer bifurcates with one portion attaching to the fibular head (F) and the anterior half passing behind (medial to) the ligament and attaching to the tibia (T). Both attach to the knee joint capsule.

the medial head of the gastrocnemius and the semimembranosus and cause a swelling behind the knee that may be considered a popliteal bursa.[31,32]

The function of the bursa is essentially plantar flexion of the foot and ankle, but by passing over the popliteal fossa, the bursa acts as a flexor and stabilizer of the knee joint. When the leg is not weight-bearing, the gastrocnemius muscle acts to flex the knee; when it is weight-bearing, the knee can be extended by the gastrocnemius muscle (Fig. 1–43). Without the effect of quadriceps, the knee can be fully extended and the leg can be stable and weight-bearing through gastrocnemius action and reliance on the posterior ligaments of the knee joint. The foot fixed to the floor, rather than the insertion of the gastrocnemius, now becomes the *origin*, and the muscle now pulls the leg backward (extension). The posterior capsule and ligaments now stabilize the knee. The lower leg can also be assisted by extending the hip and allowing the body to *lean* against the ilioinguinal Y ligament of Bigelow (Fig. 1–44).

Below and under the origin of the soleus muscle, the origin of three

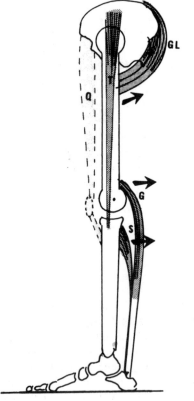

Figure 1–43. Standing balance. With non-functioning quadriceps, stance is possible by ligamentous support (the posterior popliteal capsule and anterior [hip joint capsule] Y ligament of Bigelow) and by gastrocnemius action. In the weight–bearing position, the gastrocnemius can be considered to originate from the calcaneus and insert the upper tibia and distal femur, thus extending the knee.

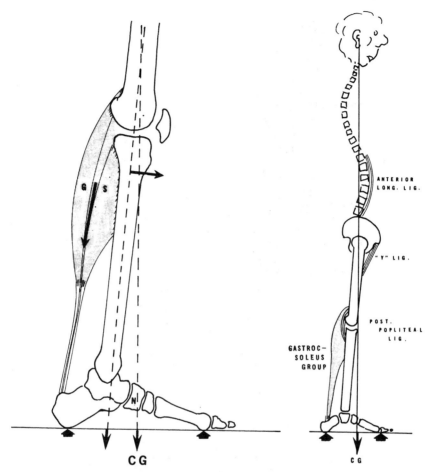

Figure 1–44. Static spine support. The relaxed person leans on his ligaments: the iliofemoral ligament (Y ligament of Bigelow), the anterior longitudinal ligament, and the posterior knee ligaments. The ankle cannot be "locked," but by leaning forward only a few degrees, the gastrocnemius must contract to support the entire body. Relaxed erect posture is principally ligamentous with only the gastrocnemius-soleus muscle group active.

bipennate muscles—the tibialis posterior, the flexor digitorum longus, and the flexor hallucis longus—are located. These muscles do not affect the knee.

BURSAE

Bursae are normally located at sites of moving tissue to permit friction-free action and diminish attrition and inflammation of these contigu-

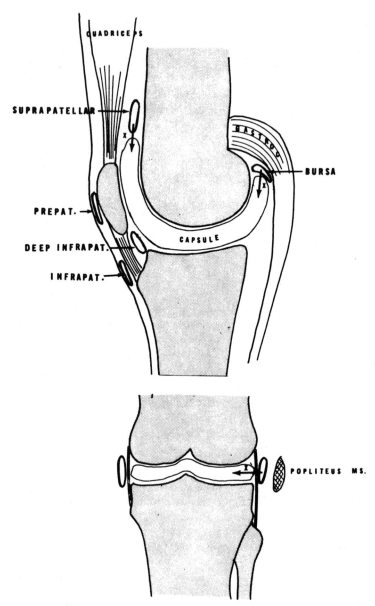

Figure 1–45. Bursae about the knee. Bursae noted: *Suprapatellar*, also termed the quadriceps femoral bursa, may communicate with the knee capsule; *Prepatellar*, between the skin and patella; *Infrapatellar* (superficial), between the skin and infrapatellar ligament; *Deep Infrapatellar*, between infrapatellar ligament and tibia; and bursae between the lateral head of the gastrocnemius and the joint capsule, the fibular collateral ligament and the biceps or popliteal tendon, and the popliteal tendon and the lateral femoral condyle. X indicates possible communication with the joint capsule.

ous tissues. There are 11 or more bursae in the region of the knee joint (Fig. 1–45). Three communicate with the knee joint: quadriceps (suprapatellar), popliteus, and the medial gastrocnemius. Three are related to the patella and the patellar tendon: prepatellar, superficial infrapatellar, and the deep infrapatellar. Two relate to the semimembranosus tendons: one, which communicates with the gastrocnemius bursa or the knee joint, or both, lies between the semimembranosus tendons and the gastrocnemius tendon, and the other lies between the semimembranosus tendon and the tibial condyle.

Two bursae lie superficially to the collateral ligaments: one between the fibular collateral ligament and the overlying biceps tendon and the other between the tibial collateral ligament and the three overlying tendons of the pes anserinus (the sartorius, gracilis, and semitendinosus). One bursa exists between the superficial and the deep parts of the tibial collateral ligaments. Irritation, inflammation, and infection of these bursae must be considered in the differential diagnosis of knee pain.

A pain in the posterior knee frequently can present itself; its causation and exact area are not always clear. This is the so-called Baker's cyst. Numerous posterior bursal inflammations are so termed. These may include bursitis between the medial head of the gastrocnemius and the semimembranosus tendon, which may communicate with the capsule space; a synovial cyst of the semitendinosus tendon; or more important may resemble a cyst and instead be an aneurysm of the popliteal artery, an A-V fistula, or a soft tissue tumor. Proper diagnosis frequently is followed by exploratory or curative surgery.

REFERENCES

1. Cailliet, R: In Mechanics of Joints. Arthritis and Physical Medicine, vol II, Ed. Sidney Licht, Waverly Press, Baltimore, 1969, pp. 17–34.
2. MacConnaill, MA: Studies in the mechanics of synovial joints. Irish J Med Sci 21: 223, 1946.
3. MacConnaill, MA: The movement of bones and joints. J Bone Joint Surg 32B:244, 1950, and 33B:251, 1951.
4. Walker, PS and Erkman, MJ: The role of the menisci in force transmission across the knee. Clin Orthop 109:184, 1975.
5. Cailliet, R: Soft Tissue Pain and Disability, ed 2. FA Davis, Philadelphia, 1988.
6. Bessette, GC and Hunter, RE: The anterior cruciate ligament. Review Article. Orthopedics 13:551, 1990.
7. Schultz, RA, et al: Mechanoreceptors in human cruciate ligaments. J Bone Joint Surg 66A:1072, 1984.
8. Zimny, ML, Schutte, M, and Dabezies, E: Mechanoreceptors in the human anterior cruciate ligament. Ann Rec 214:204, 1986.
9. Marshall, JL, et al. The anterior drawer sign: what is it? J Sports Med 3:152–158, 1975.
10. Johansson, E and Aparisi, T: Congenital absence of the cruciate ligament. Clin Orthop 162:108, 1982.
11. Noble, J: Congenital absence of anterior cruciate ligament. J Bone Joint Surg 57A:1165, 1976.

12. Tolo, VT: Congenital absence of the menisci and cruciate ligaments of the knee. J Bone Joint Surg 63A:1022, 1981.

13. Girgis, FG, Marshall, JL, and AlMonajem, ARS: The cruciate ligaments of the knee joint: Anatomical, functional and experimental analysis. Clin Orthop 106:216, 1975.

14. Marshall, JL, et al: Microvasculature of the cruciate ligaments. Phys Sports Med 7:87, 1979.

15. Sisk, TD: Traumatic affections of joints. In Edmonson, AS and Carenshaw, AH (eds): Campbells Operative Orthopaedics, Vol 1. CV Mosby, St Louis, 1980.

16. Kennedy, JC, et al: Tension studies of human knee ligaments. J Bone Joint Surg 56A:350, 1976.

17. Fu, FH, et al: Symposium: Management of Anterior Cruciate Ligament Injuries. Contemporary Orthopaedics 21:393, 1990.

18. Noyes, FR, et al: The symptomatic anterior cruciate deficient knee. I: The long term functional disability in athletically active individuals. J Bone Joint Surg 65A:154.

19. King, S, Butterwick, MA, and Cuerrier, JP: The anterior cruciate ligament: A review of recent concepts. J Orthop Sports Physical Ther 8:110, 1986.

20. Reidek, B, et al: The anterior aspect of the knee joint: An anatomical study. J Bone Joint Surg 63A:351, 1981.

21. Butler, DL, Noyes, FR, and Grood, ES: Ligamentous restraints to anterior posterior drawer in the human knee. J Bone Joint Surg 62A:259, 1980.

22. Noyes, FR, et al: Biomechanics of ligamentous failure. II. An analysis of immobilization, exercise and reconditioning effects in primates. J Bone Joint Surg 56A:1406, 1974.

23. Warren, LF and Marshall, JL: The supporting structures and layers on the medial side of the knee. J Bone Joint Surg 61A:56, 1979.

24. Brantigan, OC and Voshell, AF: The tibial collateral ligament: Its function, its bursae, and its relation to the medial meniscus. J Bone Joint Surg 25A:121, 1943.

25. Pocock, GS: Electromyographic study of the quadriceps during resistive exercises. J Am Phys Ther Assn 43:427, 1963.

26. Brewerton, JA: The function of the vastus medialis muscle. Ann Phys Med 2:164, 1955.

27. Hallen, LG and Lindahl, O: Muscle function in knee extension: An EMG study. Acta Orthop Scandinavia 38:434, 1967.

28. Lieb, FJ and Perry, J: Quadriceps function: An electromyographic study under isometric conditions. J Bone Joint Surg 53A:749, 1971.

29. Goodfellow, J, Hungerford, DS, and Zindel, M: Patellofemoral joint mechanics and pathology. J Bone Joint Surg 58B:287, 1976.

30. Basmajian, JV: Grant's Method of Anatomy, ed 8. Williams & Wilkins, Baltimore, 1971.

31. Basmajian, JV and Lovejoy, JF: Function of the popliteus muscle in man. J Bone Joint Surg 53A:557, 1971.

32. Seebacher, DB, et al: The structure of the posterolateral aspect of the knee. J Bone Joint Surg 64A:536, 1982.

CHAPTER 2

Functional Anatomy

How the knee functions determines the manner in which injury, impairment, recognition, and remedy is determined. Whereas the tibiofemoral joint appears to function as a simple hinge rotating about a fixed point on a rotating axis, the exact mechanism of knee movement is totally dissimilar.

Because of its anatomical incongruous articular surfaces, the presence of menisci, the intrinsic ligamentous structures, and the alignment of the muscular tendons, the joint is actually a complex intricate joint structure. Understanding the knee's normal functional anatomy and appreciating its deviation from normal is the basis for understanding its pathology and appreciating the appropriate remedy.

TIBIOFEMORAL MOVEMENT

Knee joint flexion or extension is a combination of rotation about a sagittal axis of the femoral condyles and a translatory gliding motion; all of this is combined with simultaneous rotation about a vertical axis. In essence, as the knee flexes, it glides in a posterior direction until it reaches the horizontal axis of rotation (flexion) (Fig. 2–1). The first 20° of flexion causes a rocking motion, then a rotating motion (Fig. 2–1). On reaching the site of axial rotation, the knee rotates (in both flexion and extension) about a longitudinal axis of the tibia. During flexion the tibia internally rotates about its own vertical axis; and during extension it externally rotates about the same axis (Fig. 2–2).

The configuration of the incongruous aspect of the articulating condylar surfaces partially causes the rotation that is observed during flexion and extension of the tibia on the femoral condyles. The difference in the length of the articulating surfaces of the medial femoral condyles and the corre-

49

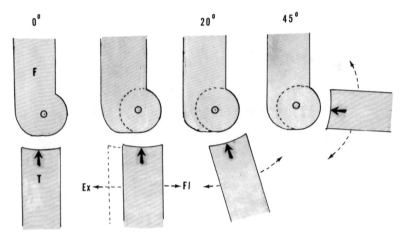

Figure 2–1. Knee flexion and extension about the femoral condyles. At full knee extension (0°) the tibia is in an anterior position. As the knee begins flexion (the first 20°) there is posterior gliding. At 20° the tibia reaches the axis of rotation and begins to rotate as depicted for 45°. The reverse occurs during extension; the beginning of extension is a rotation about the femoral condyle axis of rotation and the last degrees of extension are an anterior shear motion. Only the sagittal view is depicted in this drawing, without displaying tibial rotation.

sponding articular surface of the lateral condyles causes internal and external rotation (Fig. 2–3).

As the tibia glides on the articular surfaces of the femoral condyles in extension, the entire surface of the lateral femoral condyles is traversed. The medial condyles still have more free articular surface, thus causing the tibia to continue into external rotation (ER in Fig. 2–3). During flexion the tibia glides on the entire surface of the medial femoral condyles. When the entire surface of the lateral condyles has been traversed, the remaining free femoral medial condyle causes the tibia to glide into internal rotation (IR in Fig. 2–3). The menisci are not shown in Figure 2–3 since they are not mechanically involved in this rotatory aspect of joint motion.

LIGAMENTOUS CONTROL
OF KNEE MOTION

The medial and lateral collateral ligaments are taut at complete extension of the knee, permitting no varus or valgus motion and no rotation of the tibia on the femur. The anterior fibers of the tibial (medial) collateral ligaments incline forward as they descend on the tibia, blocking its rotation (Fig. 2–4). After 20° of flexion the ligaments become relaxed (Fig. 2–5), permitting both gliding and axial rotation. There is rotation throughout the entire knee flexion and re-extension (see Fig. 2–2), but the degree of possible

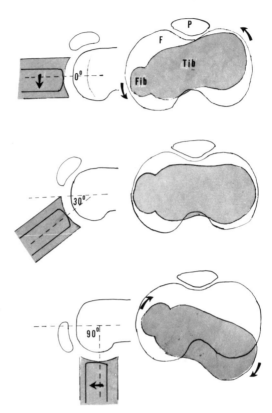

Figure 2–2. Rotation of the tibia about the femoral condyles during knee flexion and extension. At full knee extension (0°) the tibia is slightly externally rotated. At 30° of flexion the tibia and femoral condyles are parallel (no rotation). After 45° of flexion until full flexion, the tibia internally rotates as shown at 90° of flexion.

rotation increases as flexion increases and is maximum at full flexion. At 90° of flexion, 30° to 40° of rotation of the tibia on the femur is possible.

As the knee flexes and permits rotation, the deep collateral ligaments become more taut and, in conjunction with the cruciate ligaments, restrict the degree of rotation. The axis of rotation shifts as the tibia rotates about the femur (Fig. 2–6), which makes precise ligamentous action difficult to ascertain. As the tibia rotates on the femoral condyles, the capsule tightens and gradually mechanically compresses the femoral and tibial articular surfaces, limiting further rotation.

The cruciate ligaments that restrict anterior-posterior glide also limit rotation of the tibia on the femur. The anterior cruciate ligament *unwinds* during the first 15° to 20° of external rotation. As further outward rotation occurs, the anterior cruciate ligament becomes more taut as it winds around the medial aspect of the lateral femoral condyle (Fig. 2–7).[1,2]

Only certain parts of the ligament are involved throughout the range of motion of the knee. The ligament is divided into the larger bulkier posterolateral band (PLB) and the smaller anteromedial band (AMB) that runs parallel to it. A part of each band is relaxed and another part is taut throughout the range of motion, but there is a part of each band that remains taut throughout the range.[1] The AMB remains taut from 70° of flexion to full

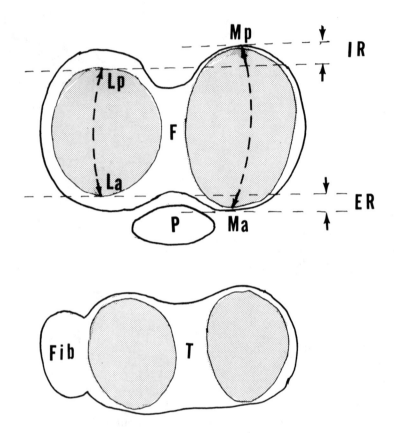

MaMp > LaLp

Figure 2–3. Articular surfaces of the femoral condyles dictating the rotatory movement of knee flexion-extension. The articular surfaces of the femoral (F) condyle and the tibial (T) facets are shaded. The patella (P) shows the anterior aspect of the knee joint.

The articulating surface distances are shown: Lp-La is the surface of the lateral femoral condyles upon which the facets of the tibia glide. The articulating surface distance of the medial femoral condyles (Mp-Ma) is longer than the lateral condylar distances (Lp-La).

The extra distance anteriorly dictates external rotation (ER) of the tibia upon the femur at the extreme of knee extension. The extra distance posteriorly of the medial condyle dictates internal rotation (IR) of the tibia upon the femur during the last degrees of knee flexion.

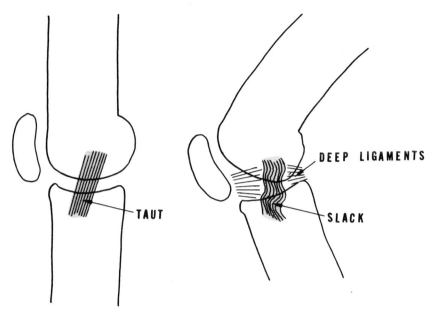

Figure 2–4. Tibial collateral ligament. (*Left*) Fully extended knee, the superficial medial ligament is oblique to alignment of leg and prevents axial rotation. (*Right*) Knee is flexed, causing ligament to become slack and allowing tibia to rotate. The deep medial ligament becomes taut and restricts rotation.

flexion and supplies 85 percent of the resistance to anterior translation at 90° flexion. The PLB is taut at full extension and until 40° to 50° of flexion. At 40° to 50° of flexion, portions of both bands are relatively relaxed and physiological anterior shear is most likely in this position.

Both internal and external rotations are limited by the anterior cruciate ligament (ACL), which provides the greatest restraint on external rotation of the tibia on the femur. Both PLB and AMB fibers restrict rotation.[2] ACL insufficiency is considered to be the most common cause of knee instability, which leads to posttraumatic osteoarthritis. The AMB and PLB are mechanical stabilizers of the knee, and they also play a large role in neuromuscular stability by being involved in sensory feedback to joint motion. The sensory role of these ligaments was suspected but has now been confirmed.[3]

The dynamic stability of the knee is dependent on the load imposed on it and the resultant reaction of the muscles about the joint. The neurological system interplay that causes this reflex neuromuscular reaction can now be ascertained. Extensive intraligamentous neural ramifications with specific nerve endings exist. These nerve endings resemble Ruffini endings, paccinian corpuscles, Golgi organlike endings at tendons, and even free fiber endings.[4] All can transmit proprioceptive impulses via the gamma-muscle spindle systems. The Ruffini endings are probably most involved because of

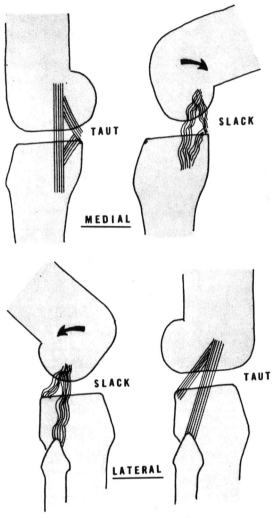

Figure 2–5. Ligamentous tautness and laxity during extension-flexion.

their characteristic threshold and rate of adoption.[5,6] The greatest number of sensory nerve endings in the cruciate ligaments is contained in the very proximal and distal portions of the ligaments.

Tension forces that act on these endings elicit appropriate reflex muscular action via the system (Fig. 2–8). Initially it was believed that extreme tractional forces acting on the tendon were needed to elicit a responsive muscular contraction. A recent study[3] has revealed that low-threshold forces initiate muscular responses.

The presence of an active spindle system innervation in the cruciate ligament indicates why surgical repair of torn anterior cruciate ligaments,

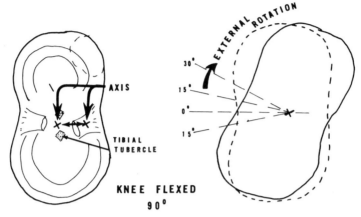

Figure 2–6. Axis of gliding and rotation. As the femur glides upon the tibia, the axis of axial rotation shifts. The degree of axial rotation varies according to the degree of flexion. None (0°) is possible at full extension or complete hyperflexion. Gradual rotation is possible until 90° of flexion is reached: 30° to 40° of rotation is possible at this point of flexion with more external rotation than internal.

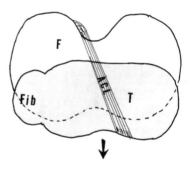

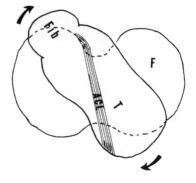

Figure 2–7. Limitation to rotation by the anterior cruciate ligament. The anterior cruciate ligament (ACL) originates from the anteromedial aspect of the rim of the tibia (T) and inserts upon the posteromedial aspect of the lateral femoral condyle of the femur (F). The upper drawing shows how the anterior cruciate ligament restricts anterior shear (*drawer*) of the tibia upon the femur (*straight arrow*). The lower drawing shows how the anterior cruciate ligament restricts external rotation (*curved arrows*) of the tibia upon the femur. The fibula (Fib) reveals the lateral aspect of the knee joint.

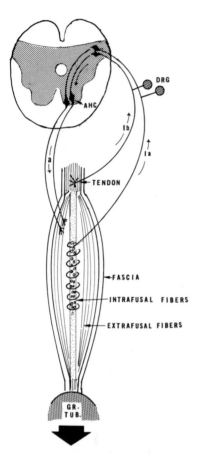

Figure 2–8. The spindle system (intrafusal fibers) is parallel with the extrafusal muscle fibers. When stretched it signals the cord by way of Ia nerve fibers (from the spindle) and Ib (from the Golgi tendon organs) through the dorsal root ganglia (DRG). An interneural connection to the anterior horn cell (AHC) causes appropriate contraction of the extrafusal muscle fibers via motor efferents. The fascia elongates according to its physiological limits. GRB in the drawing is the muscle fiber's point of attachment.

especially with replacement tissues, has been disappointing. The repaired or replaced tendon is essentially without afferent nerves, resulting in a loss of joint proprioception.

Similar proprioceptive nerves have also been found within the posterior cruciate ligament, resulting in a similar spindle system muscular reaction. Thus, both cruciate ligaments are mechanical and proprioceptive controllers of knee motion. Rehabilitation of the injured knee from cruciate ligamentous injury therefore requires not only replacement and strengthening of the remaining ligaments but also training of muscular coordination.[7]

Varus and valgus motion of the tibia on the femur, which is primarily resisted by the collateral ligaments, has been demonstrated to be excessive upon surgical sectioning of the ACL. The ACL ligament has been shown to fail at 10 percent to 15 percent elongation. Prolonged immobilization, with failure to have daily and frequent physiological elongation, causes the ligament to fail earlier and from less stress and less elongation.[8]

The posterior cruciate ligament becomes taut as the tibia glides posteriorly on the femoral condyles (Fig. 2–9). The posterior cruciate

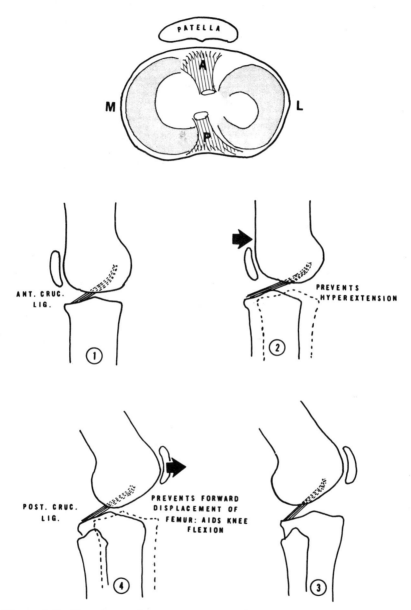

Figure 2–9. Function and restriction imposed upon cruciate ligaments. (*Top*) Superior view of the point of attachment and direction of the cruciates. Right knee medial aspect: (*1*) Direction of anterior cruciate and (*2*) method of preventing hyperextension of the knee. Right knee lateral aspect: (*3*) The posterior cruciate ligament and (*4*) manner in which it prevents forward displacement of the femur upon the tibia. By acting as a drag force it aids in normal knee flexion.

ligament arises from the posterior rim of the tibia and extends forward, upward, and inward to attach to the medial femoral condyle. In its midpassage the cruciates cross, hence the term "cruciate" (cross). During rotation of the tibia on the femur, as one of the cruciates becomes taut, the other one simultaneously relaxes. They form an axis of rotation at their site of crossing. Because of its origin and attachment, the posterior cruciate ligament prevents or limits posterior glide of the tibia on the femur.

MOTION OF THE MENISCI

The menisci are essentially attached to the tibia. The medial meniscus is attached to the medial collateral ligament around its entire periphery and at both horns via the inner connection to the spine of the tibial ligaments. The lateral meniscus at both horns is similarly attached.

If the tibiofemoral joint is anatomically considered to be the articular space within the knee, then the joint can be considered to consist of the meniscofemoral and meniscotibial spaces. This anatomical division explains the motion of the menisci (Fig. 2–10) in which the menisci move with the

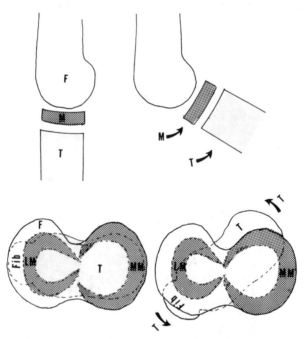

Figure 2–10. Effect of meniscal movement on knee flexion-extension and tibial rotation. The upper drawing shows the lateral view of the tibiofemoral joint divided into the meniscofemoral space and the meniscotibial space. As the knee flexes, the meniscus (*M arrow*) accompanies the tibia (*T arrow*). In the lower drawing, the menisci (LM = lateral meniscus and MM = medial meniscus) do not accompany the tibia during rotation (*T arrows*) but remain with the femoral condyles.

tibia during flexion and extension and with the femur on rotation of the flexed knee. The collateral ligamentous attachment to the menisci is responsible for this motion (Fig. 2–11).

MUSCULAR ACTION ON THE KNEE JOINT

The major muscles acting on the knee joint are the four heads of the quadriceps femoris (see Fig. 1–25). The quadriceps act in several ways: extension of the tibia on the femur, external rotation of the tibia in the last degrees of extension, and deceleration of the knee in gait. The quadriceps act on the tibia and have a direct mechanical action on the collateral ligaments of the knee, thus, maintaining their tautness.

The posterior group of muscles, predominantly the hamstring muscles (see Figs. 1–34, 1–35, and 1–36), act essentially as decelerators of the knee in gait. This is discussed in detail in Chapter 9.

The quadriceps act on the tibia because the patella has the sesamoid patella within its tendinous insertion (see Fig. 1–28). The alignment of the quadriceps as they traverse across the femur is termed the "Q angle," which is also the angle between the resultant vector of the quadriceps and the line of pull of the ligamentous patellae. The angle is determined by drawing two lines: one from the anterior-superior iliac spine through the midpoint of the patella and another line from the tibial tubercle through the midpoint of the patella (Fig. 2–12).

The direction of action of the quadriceps femoris group and the identity of the four components that act during the entire extension have been debated; the controversy is being resolved. The last 15° of extension are the most important for the stability of the knee joint. It has been determined that 60 percent more strength is needed by the quadriceps to effect these last degrees of extension. It was originally considered that the vastus medialis was the extension muscle group that was responsible for these last degrees of extension as they were the most apparent in showing atrophy after knee pathology and the last to recover during rehabilitation.

The vastus medialis acts throughout the entire range of extension[9] and not just in the last 15°. DePalma[10] stated, however, that the vastus medialis did contract more strongly in these last degrees of extension. It is now considered that the horizontal alignment of the vastus medialis prevents the patella (Fig. 2–13) from sliding laterally, which would be explained by the Q angle of quadriceps pull.

The fact that the vastus medialis appears to be the first significant muscle to atrophy after knee injury has been studied by Lieb and Perry.[11] They claim that there is general weakness of the entire quadriceps group, but the atrophy is more apparent in the vastus medialis since it is markedly oblique and very superficial and has little overlying subcutaneous fatty tissue and thin fascia.

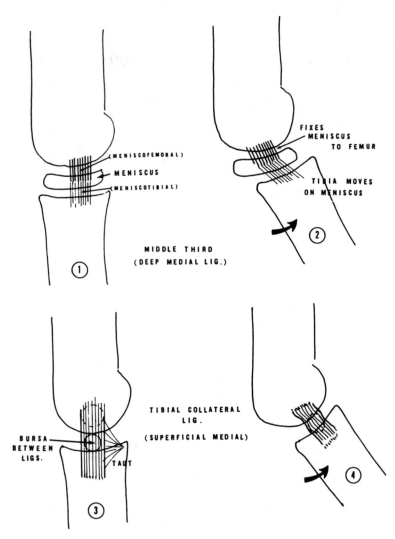

Figure 2–11. Deep medial and superficial collateral ligamentous action. The middle segment of the deep medial capsular ligament is divided into (*1*) a superior portion that fixes the medial meniscus to the femur during flexion and (*2*) an inferior portion that is slack and permits the meniscus to move. Joint spaces called meniscofemoral and meniscotibial are arbitrarily formed. (*3* and *4*) The relationship of a bursa to the superficial and deep medial ligaments is shown.

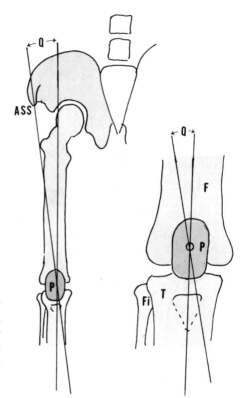

Figure 2–12. Q angle. The Q angle is designated to quantitate the direction of quadriceps pull upon the patella. The angle (Q) is formed by two lines: one drawn from the anterior superior spine (ASS) of the ilium through a midpoint on the patella (P). The other line is a vertical line drawn from the tibial condyle through a midpoint on the surface of the patella. F = femur; T = tibia; and Fi = fibula.

Inhibition of extension from pain[12] has also been stressed as evidence for quadriceps involvement. The proposal that pain inhibits active quadriceps contraction, causing gradual weakness and ultimate atrophy, has been modified and clarified. Laboratory studies that document inhibition of quadriceps contraction as the result of this pain have revealed that no reflex muscular contraction occurred when there was traction applied to normal (albeit pain-free) medial ligaments of the knee, but a reflex contraction did occur in the presence of pain from injury.[13] This reflex was inhibited by a local anesthetic. Pain was considered to initiate the reflex contraction. Apprehension caused by the pain probably initiates a reluctance to contract the quadriceps muscle with joint movement, resulting in atrophy (as opposed to atrophy from a reflex neurological activity). Effusion of the knee joint from injury conversely does "inhibit" muscular activity of the quadriceps, allegedly from reflex inhibition.[14]

These factors of inhibition and excitation play a major role in prescribing weight-bearing and non-weight-bearing exercises for the injured knee.[15] Weight-bearing exercises initiated in an injured painful knee may aggravate

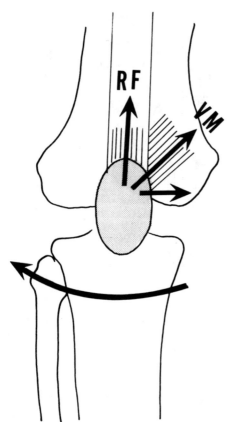

Figure 2–13. Vastus medialis function. The vastus medialis (VM) assists the quadriceps femoris (RF) in elevating the patella and extending the knee. It also pulls the patella medially to align its movement and limits external rotation of the tibia (*curved arrow*).

the pain, increase effusion, and cause instability from ligamentous stress. This resultant effusion affects the reflex, thus decreasing muscular contraction.

Non-weight-bearing exercises can reverse swelling, effusion, and pain and prevent muscular weakness and atrophy, especially when these exercises are performed against resistance.[16] Therefore, the prescription of exercise should adhere to physiological principles and begin with "setting" (isometric), then active assisted, active, and ultimately resisted exercise. Exercise is discussed under specific knee pathologies and their management.

The relation of the patellofemoral joint to injury and disease is discussed in Chapter 5, but some aspects of the functional anatomy of this joint are considered here. The alignment of the patella within the femoral fossa results in clinical pathology and impairment, as first described by Galen (129–200 AD), yet the significance of "abnormal" alignment remains controversial. Many surgical procedures have been postulated to "correct" malalignment with varying results.[17]

Factors that influence patellar position[18] and that may implicate the ligamentous tissues can be discovered by a meaningful examination. Eliciting laxity or limitation of the patellar ligaments reveals a meaningful soft tissue component. In a reported study,[17] 69 percent of patients that were examined had "hypermobility" of the patella, but its clinical significance was not ascertained. Limited transverse (mediolateral) flexibility caused by, for example, constricted medial parapatellar tissue has also been studied to determine whether its presence is required to make a decision regarding a surgical release. In addition to numerous tests for flexibility or restriction of parapatellar tissues, these authors[18] also evaluated the Q angle with the knee flexed to 90° (the "tubercle sulcus angle") as compared to the Q angle of the extended knee.

The tubercle sulcus angle is determined with the patient seated; the knee is placed at a right angle (90°) over the edge of the examining table (Fig. 2–14). The Q angle of the extended knee has been measured (see Fig. 2–13). The modified Q angle is probably more accurately measured in the seated position with the knee flexed to 90° since in this position the patella is seated within the femoral condylar groove.

A passive patellar tilt test (Fig. 2–15) has been suggested to evaluate patellar flexibility.[19] In this test, the ability of the examiner to elevate the

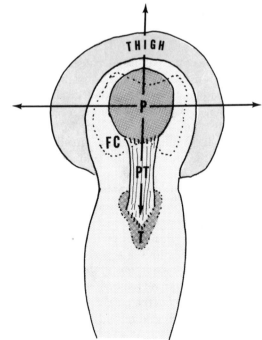

Figure 2–14. Tubercle–sulcus angle of the seated patient with knee flexed at 90°. With the patient seated and knee flexed 90°, the patellar tendon (PT) and its attachment to the tibial tubercle (T) should have a line at right angles with the horizontal line. This places the patella (P) directly under the sulcus of the femoral tubercles (FC). This is essentially a Q angle and indicates that the patella is seated centrally within the femoral condyles.

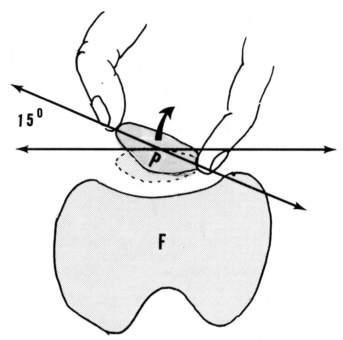

Figure 2–15. Passive patellar tilt test for parapatellar laxity. With the patient supine and the knee extended and relaxed, the patella is grasped between two fingers and tilted. Normally, approximately 15° of motion indicates normal parapatellar tissue. (Modified from Kolowich et al.)

lateral side of the patella indicates measurable soft tissue flexibility. An angle of 15° is considered within normal limits. Inability to elevate the lateral angle of the patella indicates a pathological soft tissue limitation, in this instance a limitation of the lateral tissues.

The patellar tilt test (Fig. 2–16) is done with the patient supine and the knee fully extended and the quadriceps relaxed. The patella is grasped between the fingers of the examiner, who ascertains whether the patella has remained centrally located. The degree of tilt measures the laxity of the parapatellar ligaments. A limited degree of tilt by the patella within the trochlear fossa denotes tightness or excessive laxity.

The patellar glide test (Fig. 2–16)[17] has also been advocated to determine the flexibility or limitation of the patellar soft tissues, i.e., the presence and degree of lateral or medial retinacular tightness. This test is done with the knee flexed 20° to 30° and the quadriceps completely relaxed. The degree of lateral (medial) motion is related to the amount of movement in the quadrants of the patella (see Fig. 2–16).

The lateral pull test (Fig. 2–17) measures the degree of lateral

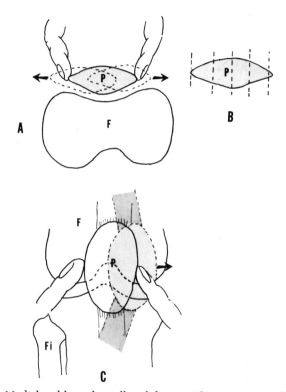

Figure 2–16. Medial and lateral patellar glide test. This passive test determines the laxity of the parapatellar tissues. The test is performed with the knee flexed 20° to 30° and completely relaxed.

(A) An overhead view of the patella (P) grasped between the examiner's fingers. F indicates the femur and the *arrows* indicate symmetrical glide. (B) The patella is divided into quadrants to quantitate the extent of movement of the patella. (C) An anterior view of the patella being moved medially (*arrow*) to test the flexibility of the lateral tissues. Fi is the fibula, indicating the lateral side of the knee joint.

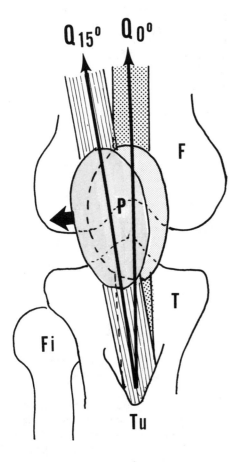

Figure 2–17. Lateral patellar pull. When there is an excessive Q angle (Q15° or more), the patella shifts laterally (*large horizontal arrow*) from a strong quadriceps contraction. With a straight quadriceps pull (Q0°, the patella remains in a vertical position from a strong quadriceps contraction.

The lines of pull are visually estimated with a line drawn from the tibial tubercle (Tu) through the center of the patella (P). F = femur; Fi = fibula; and T = tibia.

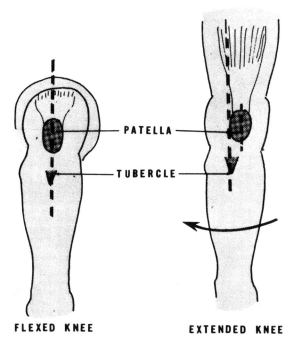

FLEXED KNEE   **EXTENDED KNEE**

Figure 2–18. Surface manifestation of tibial rotation. When the flexed knee is viewed from the front, the patella lies directly over the tibial tubercle. With the knee fully extended the tubercle is lateral to the patella, indicating external rotation during knee extension.

movement of the patella initiated by an active strong quadriceps contraction. Normally, the patella should move in a direct superior direction on contraction of the quadriceps muscle. Excessive or significant measurable lateral movement indicates an excessive Q-angle lateral pull. Direct accurate measurement by this test is difficult, but observation of lateral deviation is clear.

Tibial rotation (Fig. 2–18) must be evaluated in determining the site of the patella. The presence of significant pronation or valgus-varus deformity of the foot or ankle may also affect the position of the patella (Fig. 2–19).[18]

Medical or surgical problems of the impaired knee must be ascertained by a meaningful examination to be a deviation from normal. The significance of these abnormal findings must be considered in reaching a functional diagnosis. A meaningful diagnosis becomes mandatory in advocating a specific treatment program be it conservative or surgical.

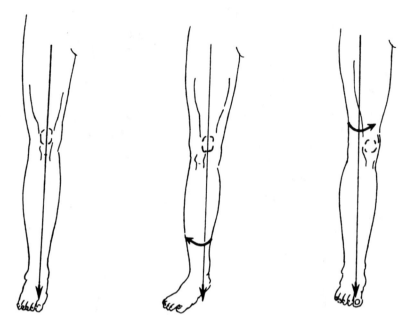

Figure 2–19. Tibial and femoral torsion. The figure to the left shows the "normal" leg in which a plumb line transects the patella and touches the foot between the first and second toes. The middle figure depicts external torsion of the leg with the tibial tubercle being externally placed to the plumb line. The figure on the right depicts internal femoral torsion.

REFERENCES

1. King, S, Butterwick, DJ, and Cuerrier, JP: The anterior cruciate ligament: A review of recent concepts. J Orthop Sports Phys Therap 8:110, 1986.
2. Bessette, GC and Hunter, RE: Review article: The anterior cruciate ligament. Orthopedics 13:551, 1990.
3. Johansson, H, Lorentzon, P, and Sojka, P: The anterior cruciate ligament: A sensor acting on the gamma-muscle-spindle systems of muscles around the knee joint. Neuro-Orthopedics 9:1, 1990.
4. Schmidt, RF: Somatovisceral Sensibility. In Schmidt, RF (ed): Fundamentals of Sensory Physiology. Springer-Verlag, New York, 1987, p 80.
5. Barrack, RL, Skinner, HB, and Buckley, SL: Proprioception in the anterior cruciate deficient knee. Amer J Sports Med 17:1, 1989.
6. Freeman, MAR and Wyke, B: The innervation of the knee joint. An anatomical and histological study. J Anat 101:505, 1967.
7. Mulder, T and Hulstyn, W: Sensory feedback therapy and theoretical knowledge of motor control and learning. Amer J Phys Med 63:226, 1984.
8. Noyes, FR, et al: Biomechanics of ligamentous failure. II. An analysis of immobilization, exercise and reconditioning in primates. J Bone Joint Surg 56A:1406, 1974.
9. Basmajian, JV, Harden, TP, and Regenos, EM: Integrated actions of the four heads of quadriceps femoris: An electromyographic study. Anat Rec 172:15, 1971.
10. DePalma, AF: Diseases of the Knee: Management in Medicine and Surgery. JB Lippincott, Philadelphia, 1954.

11. Lieb, FJ and Perry, J: Quadriceps function: An anatomical and mechanical study using amputated limbs. J Bone Joint Surg 50A:1535, 1968.
12. Hallen, LG and Lindahl, O: Muscle function in knee extension: An EMG study. Acta Orthop Scand 38:434, 1967.
13. Petersen, I and Stener, B: Experimental evaluation of the hypothesis of ligamento-muscular protective reflexes. III. A study in man using the medial collateral ligament of the knee joint. Acta Physiol Scand (Suppl 166)48:51, 1959.
14. DeAndrade, JR, Grant, C, and Dixon, A StJ. Joint distension and reflex muscle inhibition in the knee. J Bone Joint Surg 47A:313, 1965.
15. Basmajian, JV: Reeducation of vastus medialis: A misconception (Editorial). Arch Phys Med Rehab: 234, 1970.
16. DeLorme, TL: Restoration of muscle power by heavy-resistance exercises. J Bone Joint Surg 27:645, 1945.
17. Hughston, JC, Walsh, WM, and Puddu, G: Patellar Subluxation and Dislocation. WB Saunders, Philadelphia, 1984.
18. Kolowich, PA, et al: Lateral release of the patella: Indications and contraindications. Amer J Sports Med 18:359, 1990.
19. Cailliet, R: Foot and Ankle Pain. FA Davis, Philadelphia, 1983.

CHAPTER 3

Meniscus Injuries

The function of menisci has remained controversial over the decades, but more recently there has been a more gradual acceptance of the idea that they have a role in knee function. There now appears to be overwhelming evidence that the menisci play a role in load bearing, stability, and especially lubrication.[1]

Menisci performance is related to mechanical knee function, and impairment of related knee functions leads to pathology of the menisci. Menisci assist in weight bearing since they are essentially a hydrodynamic structure and are thus compliant in load bearing and impact repulsion.

Their role in knee stability is to fill the space between contiguous bone articular surfaces (Fig. 3–1). Their articular presence distracts the opposing articular surface of the femur and tibia, and causes resultant tension of the capsule and periarticular ligaments.

The role of menisci in lubrication, which is considered their major function, is to convert an incongruous joint into a more congruous one (Fig. 3–2). The alternating compression and relaxation induces the menisci to exude synovial fluid and mucin,[2] thus improving lubrication.

The functional anatomy of the knee was discussed fully in Chapter 2 but a review is warranted to gain a further understanding of the mechanopathology of meniscal injuries.[3] All knee motions are complex since flexion and extension involve gliding, simultaneous rotation, and some lateral shear. During all this, the menisci must simultaneously fulfill their mission of load bearing, stability, and lubrication.

Through its range of motion from 0° (full extension) to 140° of full flexion, the knee does not act as a simple hinge joint. At full extension the condyles of the tibia and femur interlock, allowing only 6° to 8° of internal or external rotation and medial lateral flexion. At 90° of flexion, internal and external

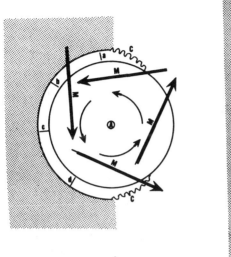
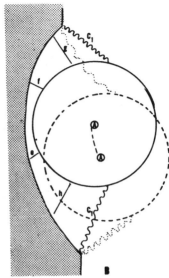

A   **B**

Figure 3–1. Congruous-incongruous joints. (A) In a congruous joint, the concave and convex surfaces are symmetrical. The articular surfaces are equidistant from each other at all points along their circumference (a = b = c = d, etc). In rotation, movement occurs about a fixed axis (A). Muscular action (M) is that of symmetical movement about this fixed axis and is needed for motion, not stability. The depth of the concave surface gives the joint stability. The capsule (C) has symmetrical elongation. (B) Incongruous joints have asymmetrical articulatory surfaces. The concave surface is elongated and the convex surface is more circular, thus the distance between them varies at each point (g>f>e<h). As the joint moves, the axis of rotation (A) shifts, and joint movement is that of gliding rather than rolling. Therefore, muscles must slide the joint and simultaneously maintain stability. The capsule varies in its elongation at all levels of movement. The glenohumeral joint is an incongruous joint.

rotation varies from 0° to 40°. At 30° of flexion, some 15° of abduction and adduction is possible.

The "functional" length of the femoral medial condyle is approximately 1.7 cm longer than that of the lateral condylar. This difference allows for the "screw home" rotation of full extension and full flexion rotation. The lateral femoral condyle literally "runs out of condyle" on which to glide in the sagittal direction and thus ends up with the medial condyles rotating along the remaining cartilage surface. In essence, during the last degrees of knee extension, the femur rotates internally while the tibia rotates externally.

The sagittal plane of the medial femoral condyle is tilted 22° to "open" the width of the articulation posteriorly. The medial tibial plateau has a greater diameter than the lateral plateau and is mostly concave, while the lateral tibial plateau is essentially flat (or even slightly convex). This

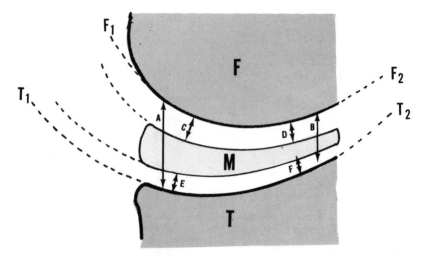

Figure 3–2. Hydrodynamic lubrication. Nonparallel joint surfaces form a wedge-shaped lubricating fluid, some of which stays at the apex. The lubricating fluid moves in layers—a, b, c, d, e—at the same speed as the articulating bone, but a layer (a–e) adheres to both articular surfaces. A shearing force between layers causes deformation of the fluid. The lubricant is both adhesive and viscous, being coated by hyaluronic acid, which is created by the synovium and cartilage. Even without movement a layer(s) remains between the two opposing joint surfaces.

incongruity enhances the potential instability of the knee joint and is amply compensated for by the menisci (see Fig. 3–2).

The cartilage coating the medial tibial plateau is three times thicker than the lateral cartilage, thus the medial component of the knee joint is capable of absorbing more impact.

The medial meniscus is C-shaped, being larger in diameter than the lateral meniscus, and its anterior horn is thinner and narrower than the posterior horn. The anterior horn is attached anteriorly to the intercondylar eminence and is thus anterior to the attachment of the anterior horn of the lateral meniscus. A transverse band passes to attach to the anterior horn of the lateral meniscus. The posterior horn of the medial meniscus is attached between the intercondylar eminence and posterior cruciate ligament. The entire outer border of the medial meniscus is firmly attached to the tibia by a thick coronary ligament. The medial meniscus is literally "firmly bound" to the tibial plateau; therefore, when the tibia moves, the meniscus also moves, but only in certain directions.

The lateral meniscus is semicircular and covers 70 to 90 percent of the tibial articular cartilage. The anterior horn of the lateral meniscus is directly attached to the intercondylar eminence. The lateral meniscus is also thinner at the anterior horn than at the posterior horn, but the lateral meniscus is correspondingly thicker than the medial meniscus.

Approximately one half of the *anterior cruciate ligament* (ACL) attaches to the posterior horn of both menisci. There is a fibrous band (Barkow's ligament) connecting the posterior horn of the lateral meniscus to the anterior horn of the medial meniscus.[4] There is no connection between the periphery of the lateral meniscus and the lateral collateral ligaments of the knee, which explains the increased mobility of the lateral meniscus as compared to the medial meniscus, which is firmly attached to the medial collateral ligaments. The anterior and posterior horn attachments that provide a point of pivot are in close approximation.

Since the lateral meniscus has greater mobility (because it does not move specifically with the tibia), it is less frequently torn. However, since the lateral meniscus is thicker than the medial meniscus, the lateral meniscus has more compression injuries.

MENISCOFEMORAL LIGAMENTS

The previously discussed ligamentous attachments are essentially attachments to the tibia. There are two ligaments that attach the menisci to the femur: the posterofemoral ligament of Wrisberg (also known as the third cruciate ligament of Robert) and the anterior meniscofemoral ligament of Humphrey.

The former ligament runs obliquely behind the posterior cruciate ligament to attach posteriorly and inferiorly to the origin of the posterior cruciate ligament. The latter ligament lies in front of the posterior cruciate ligament and inserts below the origin of the posterior cruciate ligament.[5] Meniscofemoral ligaments are found in 76 percent, 35 percent have the anterior meniscofemoral ligament of Humphrey, 35 percent the posteriofemoral ligament of Wrisberg, and 6 percent have both. These ligaments apparently work in concert with the popliteus muscle to maintain stability (by making the lateral meniscus congruent with the lateral femoral condyles).

Functionally, the meniscofemoral ligaments tighten when the femur rotates externally, while the popliteus muscle contracts to pull the meniscus back and avoid crushing forces. During normal knee action, the menisci perform their physiological function but traction and compression injuries are prevented by the ligamentous structure and the "function" of the ligaments of the knee. Injury to knee ligaments increases the likelihood of meniscal trauma.

Popliteus Muscle Function

The popliteus does not function as a knee flexor yet is vital in knee flexion as an external rotator of the femur (an internal rotator of the tibia).

The muscle "unlocks" the knee as flexion is initiated. It is most active in the first 20° to 40° of flexion as the tibia rotates medially (internally).[6] This muscle medially rotates the tibia and pulls the lateral meniscus posterolaterally.

Ligamentous Support

The anterior portion of the medial collateral ligament becomes taut in flexion, and the posterior portion becomes taut in extension. The menisci move backward in flexion and move anteriorly in extension. The menisci move in the same direction as the tibia, with the medial collateral ligament preventing anterior motion during knee extension. The semimembranosus muscle assists the popliteus muscle in pulling the lateral meniscus back during flexion and rotation of the knee.

While the medial collateral ligament is directly attached to the medial meniscus, the lateral collateral ligament is not directly attached to the lateral meniscus. The lateral collateral ligament relaxes during knee flexion and stabilizes the knee against varus forces.

Meniscus Motion

In knee extension the menisci move anteriorly and medially. In flexion the menisci move posteriorly and laterally. In flexion and extension the menisci move with the tibia on the femur. In knee rotation the lateral meniscus moves as much as 15° to 20° and moves with the femur on the tibia.

The fiber structure and orientation of the menisci[7] are both parallel and circumferential. Their direction appears to be related to the direction of motion of the tibia on the femur, which prevents tearing under physiological stresses.

Vascular Supply

The vascular supply originates from the genicular branches, which penetrate from the periphery of the menisci a distance of 1 to 3 mm within a synovial "fringe." Before regeneration of a damaged meniscus can occur, the synovial fringe on the outer third of the meniscus must heal. Studies on meniscal injuries in dogs[8] found that healing never occurs, except with scar tissue, if the meniscal tear communicates with the peripheral portion of the meniscus. Tears occurring in the periphery do heal with pseudocartilage, which contains no cartilaginous cells. Tears within the middle portion of the menisci do not heal.

Other Mechanical Aspects

The lubrication of the knee joint, which has been in part attributed to the presence of the menisci, is dependent on the congruity of the joints[9] (Fig. 3–2) and on hydrodynamic lubrication (Fig. 3–3). The motion of two opposing surfaces separated by a viscous fluid creates pressures of equal magnitude at each surface.[10] In the knee, as in any incongruous joint, lubrication occurs through one film layer gliding on the other, which keeps the surfaces of the joints apart yet lubricated.

Before discussing meniscal pathology and clinical manifestations, we must discuss other mechanical aspects of knee function and related meniscal function. The menisci separate the femoral condyles from the tibial plateau and thus make taut the ligaments stabilizing the joint. This is confirmed by the fact that a meniscectomy causes the joint space to narrow radiologically.[11]

With the knee extended, the weight-bearing contact of the medial side is 1.6 times greater than that of the lateral side[12] but as the knee flexes past 30°, the amount of weight bearing decreases. At heel strike in normal gait, the force of impact is approximately four times that of the body weight and, being borne on the extended knee, is impressed on the greatest area of articular contact.

As the gait proceeds to the stance phase[13] (Fig. 3–4), the knee flexes approximately 40° and the impact force diminishes to two times that of the body weight. The quadriceps has acted to ensure that the knee is extended

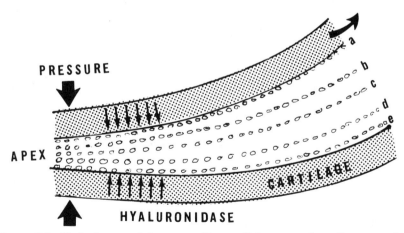

Figure 3–3. Hydrodynamic lubrication. Nonparallel joint surfaces form a wedge-shaped lubricating fluid, some of which stays at the apex. The lubricating fluid moves in layers—a, b, c, d, e—at the same speed as the articulating bone, but a layer (a–e) adheres to both articular surfaces. A shearing force between layers causes deformation of the fluid.

The lubricant is both adhesive and viscous, being coated by hyaluronic acid, which is created by the synovium and cartilage. Even without movement a layer(s) remains between the two opposing joint surfaces.

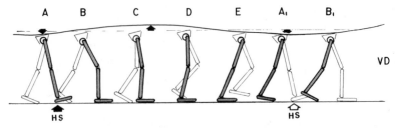

Figure 3–4. Determinants of gait. From A, which is the heel-strike (HS) position of the swing phase, the knee gradually flexes to maintain a level vertical elevation and depression of the pelvis (*line with black arrows*). Therefore, the gait requires less energy expenditure. The knee re-extends as E (heel-off position) approaches. A_1 depicts the next phase of the heel strike of the other leg.

and the leg is flexed at the hip in the swing-through phase (Fig. 3–5). As midstance approaches, the quadriceps contracts to support the knee that has been flexed to 40° at the onset and through the midstance phase. The knee gradually "locks" on its ligaments in extension in the heel-off and toe-off phases. During this phase the quadriceps is inactive. Studies of the knee during gait have estimated that 50 percent of the impact is absorbed by the menisci.[14]

PATHOMECHANICS OF MENISCAL INJURIES

The precise role of the menisci in the normal movement of the femur on the tibia has been debated for decades. Some clinicians believed that the menisci are useless, while others believed that they are a vital component. The accepted role of the meniscus has been determined by engineering studies and from evaluations of knees that have had partial or total removal of their menisci. The current concept is that menisci are vital for weight bearing, conversion of incongruous joint surfaces into congruous surfaces, stability, and lubrication.

The advent of arthroscopy and arthroscopic surgical intervention is helping to answer the following questions: What are the mechanical factors that cause meniscal injury? How are these injuries repaired? What are the symptoms of injury and how they are best treated?

Injury to the menisci is considered to result from traction, compression, or torque forces or from a combination of all three. Injuries occur mainly from entrapment of the menisci between the femoral heads and the tibial plateau when either a severe external force exceeds the normal alignment of the joint components or when there is entrapment between the femur and tibia from an unphysiological movement.

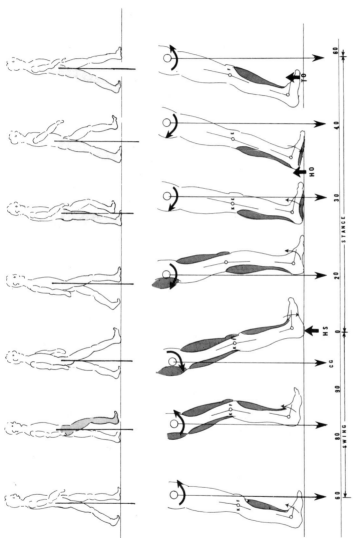

Figure 3–5. Quadriceps function in gait. As the leg enters the swing phase (60), the quadriceps extends the knee and flexes the hip. The knee is initially slightly bent (80) until the heel strike (0 and HS).

As the body glides forward on the leg stance, the knee flexes 40° (20). The quadriceps supports the weight, but as the body passes midstance (30), the knee locks in extension on its ligaments and the quadriceps relaxes. The knee remains extended at heel off (HO) and toe off (TO) to enter another swing phase. There is rotation of the tibia on the femur during these phases, but this is not represented in the illustration.

The normal flexion and extension of the knee is dictated by the shape and curvatures of the opposing condylar surfaces of the femur and the tibia. Motion is guided and limited by ligamentous and muscular forces that operate on the femur and tibia as well as on the menisci. In normal knee function, the two opposing articular cartilaginous surfaces remain sufficiently separated to offer room for the two menisci. When the joint no longer offers this adequate space, compression of the menisci results.

The menisci move with the tibia and femur during flexion and extension and the associated rotation. This movement is well coordinated because each meniscus is connected to the femur and tibia by ligaments that ensure the menisci are present in the proper zone of the joint space during all physiological movements. Normal physiological movement is assured by proper muscular action and by ligamentous structures that always keep the menisci in the right place at the right time. Only when this fails to occur does injury to the menisci occur.

The offending forces may be internal or external. An example of an internal force is the inappropriate knee extension suffered by an athlete who, in the performance of an athletic activity, wears spiked shoes that grip the foot to the surface. The expected external rotation during the last degrees of extension causes internal rotation. The femoral condyle "crushes" the meniscus on the tibial plateau as the joint space narrows (Fig. 3–6). Another example of an internal injury can occur in a person in a marked knee-flexed, squat position who rises rapidly while the feet remain fixed to the surface, thus impeding adequate rotation during extension.

An example of external force is a violent blow to the knee. The blow may hit the knee from the side, causing severe varus or valgus (Fig. 3–7), or from the front or rear, causing either hyperextension or hyperflexion. Any of these forced motions of the knee pushes the condyle on the tibial plateau and entraps the enclosed meniscus.

The mechanism of injury is elicited from a spectator or the injured athlete. The clinician then reconstructs the injury and its mechanical impact on the meniscus and whether there was any injury to the ligaments.

The differential diagnoses of meniscal tears are numerous and are usually ascertained retrospectively from clinical, radiological, or especially arthroscopic evaluation of the injured patient. Besides the mechanical factors that can be implicated in meniscal tears, other factors have been considered, including constitutional inadequacy, ligamentous laxity, muscular inadequacy, faulty work habits, obesity, and severe genu valgum or varum.

The injury that occurs to the meniscus is clinically termed a "tear" in that the continuity of the meniscal fibers is disrupted (Fig. 3–8).[15] The microscopic structure of the meniscus consists of three distinct zones of collagen bundles. The outer one third of the meniscus is composed of circumferential fibers. It must be noted that this area is the only portion of the meniscus that receives vascular supply. The other two zones contain

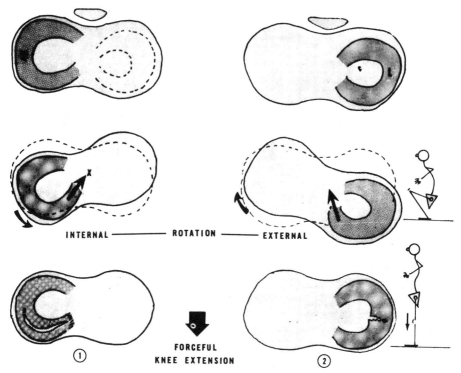

Figure 3–6. Mechanism of meniscus tear. (*1*) With the knee fully flexed and the femur *internally* rotated, the medial meniscus is displaced posteriorly and the posterior horn (X) moves toward the center. Forceful extension of the knee causes a longitudinal tearing because of the meniscus capsular attachment or tear of the posterior attachment, or both. (*2*) With the knee fully flexed and the femur *externally* rotated, the lateral meniscus is moved posteriorly and its posterior horn toward the center of the joint. Forceful knee extension *elongates* the meniscus, causing radial tearing on the medial (inner) margin of the meniscus.

fibers that run in a transverse direction. The two zones are divided into a superior and an inferior bundle by a thin, albeit thickened, bundle called the *middle perforating bundle* (MPB in Fig. 3–8). There are also vertical fibers within the two inner transverse bundle fibers that allegedly act as stabilizers of the meniscus. They are not shown in the figure.

Tearing of the meniscus causes symptoms and impairment. Symptoms occur because the meniscus is damaged and is no longer smooth; thus, it cannot mold itself to the opposing articular surfaces or remain in its proper position during joint motion. The new, irregular contour of the meniscus prevents its motion within the joint space, although the joint still moves physiologically and remains adequately open.

The site, direction, and extent of the tear within the meniscus can vary

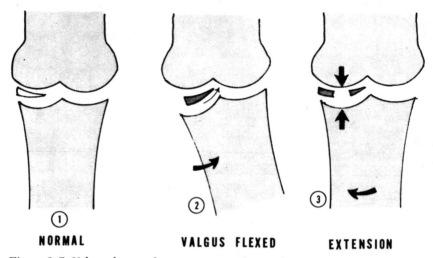

NORMAL   **VALGUS FLEXED**   **EXTENSION**

Figure 3–7. Valgus theory of meniscus tear. The combination of knee flexion with forced valgus, which opens the medial aspect of the knee joint, plus the deeper, more concave tibial condyle, forces the meniscus toward the center of the joint. Re-extension pinches the entrapped meniscus between the opposing condyles.

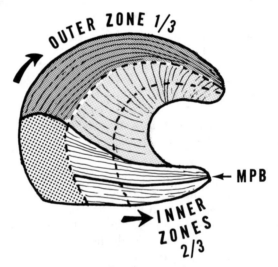

Figure 3–8. Microscopic structure of a meniscus. The meniscus is divided into three zones, each having two layers. The outer zone has circumferentially placed collagen fibers, and the two inner layers have collagen fibers that run radially (transverse zone). Each inner layer is divided into two layers by a thin, yet thickened, layer of fibers termed the *middle perforating bundle* (MPB). (Modified after Voto and Ewing.[15])

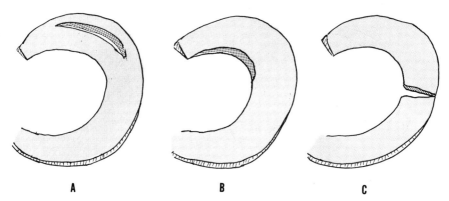

Figure 3–9. Major types of meniscal tears. (*A*) A circumferential (longitudinal) tear. (*B*) A horizontal tear that essentially divides the meniscus into superior and inferior layers. These tears can convert into flaps. (*C*) A radial (transverse or oblique) tear.

(Fig. 3–9).[16] The tear may be in an innocuous site with no disruption of the precise contours of the meniscus, which causes no symptoms. The tear may be longitudinal (see Fig. 3–9A), which allows the inner zone to spread from the inner zone, thus causing the inner zonal area to be larger (relatively thicker) than is permitted by the allotted joint space. The tear may be horizontal (Fig. 3–10), causing the inner zone to become thicker in that area. The tear may also be in a radial direction (see Fig. 3–9C and transverse in Fig. 3–10).

A specific nomenclature has been suggested[15] (Fig. 3–10) for specifying the exact site of tear in the meniscus. This nomenclature is obviously used after arthrostomy or arthroscopy, retrospectively linking the site and type of tear with the symptomatology and clinical findings. The areas have been numbered 1 through 9 and are the designation of the author without, as yet, accepted universal standardization. The torn meniscus can now be designated as vertical, horizontal,[17] or transverse, with or without flap, and, if so, superior or inferior (Fig. 3–11). The length of the tear can also be indicated by the zones which are involved as well as by the remnant of meniscal attachments. Such documentation and standardization provides a meaningful descriptive nomenclature. The provoking factors, the "ideal" surgical procedure, and the prognosis can then evolve.

DIAGNOSTIC SIGNS AND SYMPTOMS

The history given by the patient is that of acute severe knee pain after an incident, "as if something tore within my knee." The incident may be a turning and twisting movement during an athletic activity or direct blow to

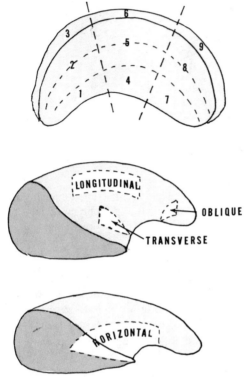

Figure 3–10. Primary tear patterns of the meniscus: recommended zoning. The upper drawing depicts a method of specific zoning to standardize the site of lesion. (Modified after Voto and Ewing.[15]) The two lower drawings illustrate the designation of direction of meniscal tears.

the knee. As previously stated, the precise incident may not be specifically recalled and may need confirmation from an observer of the event.

Pain from an acute meniscal tear usually causes immediate cessation of all activities. In a ligamentous injury without meniscal pathology, activities may frequently continue in spite of the pain and discomfort, but this rarely happens in meniscal injury.

Since pain occurs because of the liberation of nociceptor substances, such as prostaglandins, kinins, factor P, etc., that irritate the nerve endings of demyelinated nerve fibers, it must be assumed that there is, in conjunction with the meniscal tearing, some synovial inflammatory reaction. The inflamed synovium may be the synovium of the articular cartilages of the condyles or of the tibial plateaus that become irritated as a result of the "foreign body" reaction of the deformed meniscus.

Pain may be experienced as a result of the ligamentous connection of the meniscus since the meniscus is essentially aneural except possibly within a thin circumferential layer of the medial meniscus. (This has been demonstrated in studies of the outer circumferential layers of the intervertebral disc, which has a structure similar to cartilage and is considered aneural.) Central lesions and incomplete radial tears of the meniscus may be asymptomatic unless they initiate a deformation of the precise contours of the meniscus that mechanically prevents the condyles from moving without interference.

Effusion is usually present after a significant meniscal injury. The absence of effusion indicates that another type of injury must be suspected as the cause of the pain and limitation. Effusion is less frequent and less severe in injuries of the lateral meniscus than in those of the medial because of the minimal peripheral capsular attachment; however, effusion still occurs.

Hemarthrosis rather than effusion implies a more severe injury.[18] The finding of blood in the knee joint usually indicates severe injury to an internal structure. Prompt diagnosis and treatment[19] provides the best chance for functional recovery; thus an initial precise diagnosis is mandatory.

An initial diagnostic examination that rules out collateral and cruciate ligamentous tears and initial x-ray studies that rule out intra-articular fractures may diminish inappropriate concern for the significance of the injury. These tests are enumerated in Chapter 4. They can be done as an office procedure or on the field if the knee is seen early in the injury before

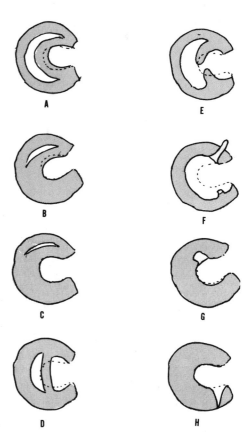

Figure 3–11. Varieties of meniscus tears. In this illustration only medial meniscus tears are shown. (A) Complete tear still attached. (B) Partial tear. (C) Partial tear remaining in situ (not probably symptomatic). (D) Partial tear encroaching into the joint. (E) Complete tear with detached fragments. (F) Complete tear in which the detached fragments form flaps that are either inferior or superior to the remaining meniscus. (G) A torn flap with the remaining meniscus intact. (H) Vertical tear with slight retraction of the remaining meniscus.

significant effusion. They are often best done under an anesthetic. A delay of 4 hours before the onset of effusion or hemarthrosis that reveals "negative" ligamentous signs frequently allays concern from the examiner. However, studies may eventually reveal that meniscal as well as ligamentous injuries have occurred.

Arthroscopic examination was originally considered contraindicated in the presence of hemarthrosis because the blood would cause limited visibility through the scope. More recently, florid irrigation of the joint preceding arthroscopic examination has changed this contraindication, and internal examination of the knee through the arthroscope has been shown to be valuable.[20] Discovery of significant injuries to ligaments, unsuspected meniscal injuries, and subchondral fractures (in spite of negative clinical signs) has made arthroscopic examination of a knee with hemarthrosis strongly indicated.[18]

Tenderness elicited along the entire knee joint line is a valuable sign if it is properly evaluated. If the medial meniscus is torn, tenderness can be elicited along the entire periphery but is most prominent along the posterior line of attachment (since this is the more prominent site of tear) rather than at the anterior aspect of the joint. A tear of a collateral ligament usually causes tenderness above or below the joint line. This is in contrast to a meniscal tear since this is where tearing of the ligament occurs most frequently.

Locking rarely occurs as a consequence of an acute meniscal tear, and when locking does occur, it may occur spontaneously with rapid, spontaneous release. Because tearing usually occurs with no displacement or bunching in the posterior one third of the meniscus (Fig. 3–11) there is no mechanical impairment of knee motion. If the tear is in the anterior aspect of the meniscus, locking may occur, that is, full extension of the knee is mechanically prevented. True locking may be sudden and unlocking may also occur suddenly. Gradual locking may result from effusion or hemarthrosis, especially within the infrapatellar fat pad (Fig. 3–12). Not all meniscal injuries have a history of locking, so it cannot be considered a cardinal diagnostic sign or complaint. A history of locking may be absent in 50 percent of confirmed meniscal tears.

The knee may buckle or "give way" during walking or jogging, especially on irregular terrain. This symptom seems more prevalent in tears of the posterior segment of the meniscus with no apparent mechanical explanation.

"Clicking" that is audible to the patient or examiner may be symptomatic of a meniscal tear, but the clicking may also be caused by an irregular femoral condyle passing over an articular irregularity in the tibial plateau, chondromalacia patellae, articular grating in a degenerative arthritis, or a hamstring tendon passing over the femoral condyle. Careful manual palpation of the site of clicking during active or passive knee flexion and exten-

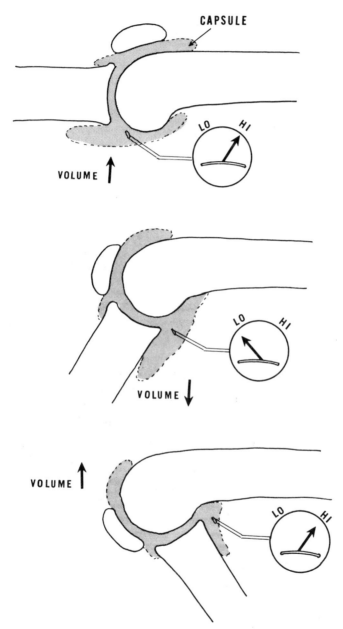

Figure 3–12. Pressure variations with knee position. With the knee in midflexed position (*middle*), there is the lowest pressure, thus less irritation of sensory (pain) and pressure nerves. This is the position assumed by the patient who avoids full extension (*top*) or further flexion (*bottom*).

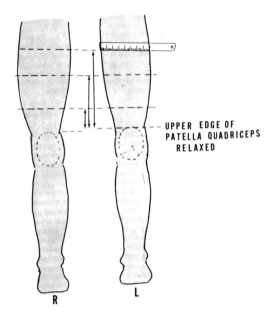

UPPER EDGE OF
PATELLA QUADRICEPS
RELAXED

R   L

Figure 3–13. Quadriceps measurement for atrophy. Comparative measurement of quadriceps circumference is done at measured distances (4, 6, 8, 10, and 12 inches) from upper edge of patella with quadriceps relaxed.

sion usually determines the site and hence the tissue responsible for the clicking.

Quadriceps atrophy occurs rapidly in a meniscal injury with resultant effusion, hemarthrosis, and/or functional impairment. Neurological reflex quadriceps inhibition resulting from effusion[21] has been confirmed experimentally. Atrophy is measurable (Fig. 3–13) within days after an injury and is most pronounced in an injury to the vastus medialis. The occurrence of isolated atrophy in the vastus medialis rather than throughout the entire quadriceps has been refuted by Lieb and Perry.[22] These authors confirmed that atrophy is generalized throughout the entire quadriceps, but atrophy is more visually apparent in the medialis since this muscle is distinctly oblique and is covered with little subcutaneous tissue; hence injury to the vastus medialis is more visible.

Clinical Meniscus Signs

The so-called meniscus signs that are to be elicited during a clinical examination and that confirm the presence of a meniscal tear are numerous and vary according to the authors who initially described them. These signs unfortunately bear the examiner's name rather than the physiological basis for the test; hence, the tests vary in their interpretations.

Most meniscal signs are an elicitation of a clicking, crepitation, limitation, or symptom produced as a result of the limitation in normal joint motion by the mechanical intrusion of the deformed meniscus. All meniscus tests use numerous passively performed knee joint motions in an attempt to determine the source of the limitation when the meniscal defect appears and restricts motion. The exact type and site of meniscal damage is allegedly discovered from these maneuvers. The adequacy of joint spacing is acknowledged during the range of motion being elicited, and the meniscus is assumed to normally allow this motion. However, when the meniscus is damaged, it becomes a "foreign body."

McMurray Test. The McMurray test is a time-honored test in which the patient is placed in the recumbent position, the leg is flexed at the hip to a right angle, and the knee is bent to form a right angle (Fig. 3–14). To test the integrity of the medial meniscus, the physician "internally" rotates the lower leg on the femur and slowly extends the leg while internal rotation is maintained. Crepitation, pain, or limitation indicates a possible tear in the medial meniscus, causing the meniscus to be deformed, hence limiting extension. The test is valid only during initial extension from 90° of flexion but does not confirm a tear in the last degrees, which would implicate a tear of the anterior horn of the meniscus. The McMurray test applies to the lateral meniscus if the lower leg is "externally" rotated on the flexed knee and then slowly and gradually extended.

Apley Test. The Apley test is similar in mechanism to the McMurray test but tries to differentiate a meniscal lesion from a capsular or ligamentous injury. In this test, the patient is placed in the prone position and the knee is flexed at a right angle (90°) (Fig. 3–15). The hip is extended to neutral, which is different from the McMurray test position.

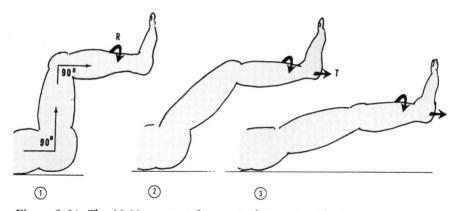

Figure 3–14. The McMurray test for meniscal integrity. The McMurray test is performed with the patient supine, hip flexed to right angle, and knee flexed to 90° (*1*). The lower leg is rotated internally to test the medial meniscus and externally to test the lateral meniscus. Grating (crepitation), resistance, and/or pain indicates possible meniscus pathology.

The knee is then gradually extended (*2* and *3*), again with simultaneous rotation. This motion—extension and rotation—should be free, with no crepitation or pain. If there is meniscal pathology, crepitation occurs as does limitation and pain. The test is not valid in the last 10° to 15° of full extension.

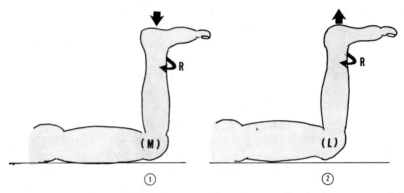

Figure 3–15. Meniscus test: the Apley test. The Apley test checks the integrity of the knee ligamentous structures and of the menisci. It is performed in two aspects. (*1*) With the patient prone and the knee flexed to a right angle, downward pressure is put upon the lower leg. The leg is then rotated to test the menisci (M). This maneuver compresses the menisci between the femoral condyles and the tibial plateau (as does the McMurray test). With the lower leg internally rotated the medial meniscus is tested. Grating, crepitation, limitation, and pain imply meniscal damage.

From the same position (2) the leg is elevated, which places traction upon the ligaments (L). Excessive motion, deduced by a comparison to the contralateral side, indicates laxity or injury to the knee ligaments and capsule.

The lower leg is flexed (at a right angle), then internally and externally rotated with simultaneous upward traction. The traction tests the integrity of the capsule and ligaments while distracting the joint and releasing any entrapment of the menisci. The test is then performed by pressing the lower leg downward, hence compressing the joint. The internal and external rotation, together with the downward pressure, allegedly compress any defect of the meniscus between the femoral condyles and the tibial plateaus, revealing any mensical deformity.

Steinmann's Test. The Steinmann test is also termed the *tenderness displacement test* (Fig. 3–16). When there is internal pathology within the knee joint, there often is tenderness that can be elicited by palpation along the joint space. Anterior meniscus pathology is supposed to cause tenderness anterior to the midline. The tenderness migrates toward the midline if there is also ligamentous or central meniscal pathology. This test is difficult to perform and interpret properly, but if there is concern about differential diagnosis, theoretically, the tenderness test "does not migrate with knee flexion" in degenerative knee articular disease.

Hyperflexion Meniscus Test. In the presence of a posterior horn meniscal tear, the hyperflexion meniscus test (Fig. 3–17) is often positive. With the patient in the prone position, the knee is hyperflexed, then passively rotated internally and externally. In this maneuver, any meniscal pathology of the posterior horn causes painful clicking when the damaged meniscus passes between the femoral condyles and the tibial plateau. The

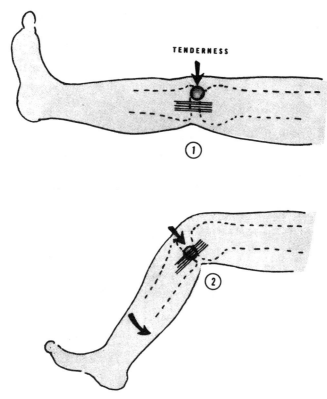

Figure 3–16. Meniscus sign: tenderness displacement test. (*1*) With the extended knee, the tenderness over the medial meniscus occurs anteriorly. (*2*) As the knee is flexed the tenderness migrates posteriorly toward the medial collateral ligament.

involvement of the medial or lateral meniscus can be determined by noting whether the internal or external rotation, respectively, causes a greater reaction.

There are many similar tests for meniscal lesions proposed in the literature, but all are founded on the mechanical basis that the deformed meniscus becomes entrapped between the moving femoral condyles and the tibial plateau. An understanding of where the meniscus should be at a particular point of extension and flexion and internal and external rotation will help determine which meniscus is involved and which portion of the meniscus is injured.

Diagnostic Tests

Arthrography. Arthrography was considered a specific test to ascertain the presence of meniscal pathology as well as its site, type, and extent of damage. Arthrography is performed by injecting dye into the joint, which outlines the contours of the intra-articular tissues (Fig. 3–18 and 3–19).

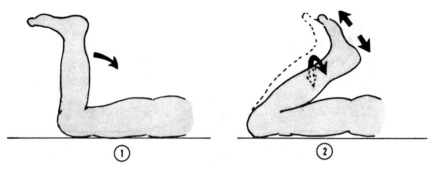

Figure 3–17. Hyperflexion meniscus test. With the patient prone, the knee is flexed to 90°. Then, with internal or external rotation of the leg upon the femur, the knee is *hyperflexed*. Painful clicking may indicate a posterior meniscus tear. Doing this maneuver may cause the knee to lock from movement of the fragment into the joint.

A careful study of an arthrogram by a well-trained radiologist or diagnostic orthopaedist has been considered to yield a reasonably accurate diagnosis. There are some aspects of the contents of the knee joint that remain obscure even with the best procedure, so its total accuracy is not assured.

Magnetic Resonance Imaging. Arthrography still has its exponents, but this test now has been largely replaced by magnetic resonance imaging (MRI). MRI has also largely replaced computerized tomography (CT) scanning, which had begun to replace arthrography. MRI is noninvasive and

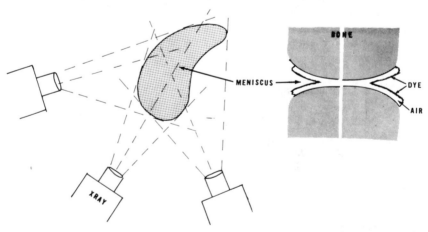

Figure 3–18. Arthrography. The knee, and thus the meniscus, is rotated before the x-ray so that both poles and the entire meniscus are visualized. (*Left*) The lateral and medial aspects of the joint are visualized separately. (*Right*) The air creates contrast and the dye coats all intra-articular tissues.

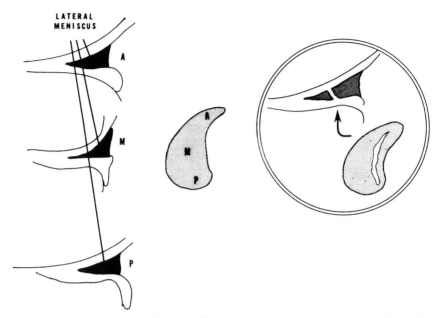

Figure 3–19. Arthrograms. (*Center*) Normal lateral menisci: A, anterior horn; M, middle horn; P, posterior horn. (*Left*) What is seen on lateral x-ray films. (*Right*) An arthrogram taken of a torn meniscus.

accurately and precisely reveals the status of the menisci in all their aspects, the condylar and plateau cartilage, and the ligaments.

The accuracy of MRI is well documented.[23] Unfortunately MRI is currently a very expensive procedure and is not available in all medical centers and even radiology departments that have this equipment may not be staffed with personnel trained to evaluate musculoskeletal MRIs. MRI is the most diagnostically accurate, noninvasive procedure of the knee today. However, it must only be used when a thorough clinical evaluation of the painful impaired knee causes the clinician to suspect significant pathology. It must not replace clinical judgment, and it must not be the sole basis for surgical intervention.

Arthroscopy. The torn meniscus has been and continues to be the most common mechanical cause of knee symptoms. Meniscectomy continues to be the most commonly performed surgical procedure to the knee. The advent and perfection of arthroscopy have revolutionized knee evaluation and treatment. Direct vision of the knee joint's contents has increased our understanding of knee conditions. The technique is time consuming and, as yet, restricted to the limited albeit increasing number of physicians who have mastered the technique. What is seen by the arthroscoper depends on her or his experience. Even as recently as 1980, few individuals in England had mastered the technique and gained the required skills[24] as compared to the United States. Since then, the number of skilled performers has increased in all countries, as judged by its increasing mention in the medical literature.

Prior to arthroscopic evaluation and surgical treatment, most procedures involved total meniscectomy, resulting in a large number of degenerative arthritic changes of the tibiofemoral cartilage. Surgery in the prearthroscopy era was based on a diagnosis obtained by a clinical evaluation and "confirmed" by arthrography. The astute orthopaedist Watson-Jones[25] advocated removing the suspected meniscus even if it was found to be normal for fear of leaving an unrecognized posterior tear. Currently, the goal of meniscal surgery should always be to preserve as much meniscus as possible after removal of the offending injured portion.

Numerous surgeons claimed that posterior meniscal tears were often visualized by arthrography. This is also a "blind" area for the arthroscope, so MRI studies are justified when this lesion is suspected. Again, a precise clinical examination must raise the possibility of a posterior horn tear. "As no specific signs or symptoms consistently mean a specific lesion, it is best, in all but the most acute and obvious case, to examine the patient two or three times over several weeks before any firm surgical decision is made."[24] This advice predates the advent of MRI, but the premise is still valid.

A small posterior tear that cannot be demonstrated is likely to be unimportant, and although the sequelae of removing the meniscus are well documented, the effect of leaving behind a small tear of the posterior meniscus remains unknown.

The amount of time that can elapse between diagnosis and removal of damaged meniscus without degenerative articular changes occurring in the condyles and plateaus varies. Some authors recommend immediate intervention,[26,27] while others recommend waiting.[28] These time factors have not yet been ascertained.

The arthroscope permits not only direct visualization of the injury but also allows the surgeon to utilize a blunt hook that may distract the torn meniscus and reveal an otherwise unnoticed tear. The "flap" of torn meniscus (Fig. 3–11F and 3–11G) is also visible and hence removable by the blunt hook.[16] Since the tear pattern significantly determines the eventual result of the surgical procedure, the pattern must be clearly ascertained.

The term "flap tear" implies that a fragment of meniscal tissue is torn along two planes and remains attached, while becoming mobile about its narrow base (Fig. 3–20). A vertical tear combines with a horizontal tear or a vertical tear combines with a transverse tear to form a flap that folds upward or downward, becoming a "foreign body" that deforms the contour of the meniscus.

In summary, the mechanics of the flap is abnormal because flexion and extension of the knee occurs between the articular surface of the femur and the upper surface of the meniscus; hence, the superior flap could cause

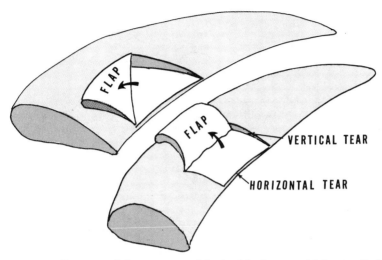

Figure 3–20. Flap tear of the meniscus. Meniscal lesions combining vertical and horizontal tears result in the formation of a flap that curls superiorly or inferiorly, depending on which region of the central meniscus is torn. The horizontal tear occurs above or below the *middle perforating bundle* (MPB) of the inner zone (see Fig. 3–8).

The base of the flap can be seen from either above or below the figure, depending on the type of the predominant tearing: vertical or horizontal. These tears are seen using arthroscopy and may be detected with MRI.

irritation. Conversely, rotation of the knee occurs between the inferior surface of the meniscus and the cartilage of the tibial plateaus; hence, the inferior flaps could also cause irritation.

In spite of improved arthroscopic examinations and reports of arthrotomies, surgical intervention has been prescribed for many normal menisci.[29–31] The arthroscopist must be aware of the limitations of surgical intervention and of the adverse consequences of iatrogenic injury to articular cartilage.[32]

Degenerative arthritis will be more thoroughly discussed in Chapter 6, but some mention of it here is warranted since this is a dreaded sequela of an inadequate amount of meniscal tissue remaining after surgical removal and of damaged meniscus remaining within the knee joint.

The structure of normal cartilage (Fig. 3–21) and the changes resulting from trauma explain the mechanism by which meniscal injury predisposes to early degenerative arthritis. The loss of the meniscus causes excessive[33] pressure on the articular cartilages of the opposing bones of the knee joint (Fig. 3–22), leading to degenerative changes. Salvaging as much meniscus as possible is the major reason for any therapy of meniscal damage.

The pathological events leading to osteoarthritis and its classification are not standardized. Grading is as follows:

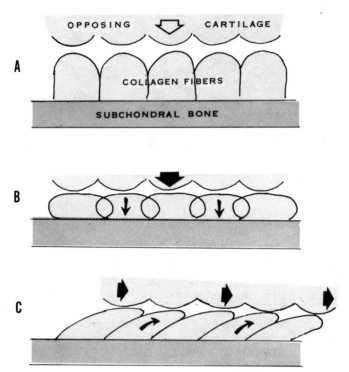

Figure 3–21. Deformation of articular cartilage. (*A*) Normal cartilage with springlike bands of collagen within a mucoid matrix are depicted. (*B*) Pressure from opposing cartilage causes the collagen fibers to compress (*small arrows*), in turn causing lubricating fluid to be released into the joint. (*C*) Translation forces cause a shear effect (*three large arrows*), deforming the fibers (*curved arrows*). If these shear forces are excessive or repetitive, they may cause deterioration of the collagen fibers, initiating the early stages of degenerative arthritis.

Grade I: There is flaking of the superficial zone with loss of collagen fibers in that zone (Fig. 3–23). The loss of continuity of the collagen fibers decreases the amount of cartilage expansion on release of the compression forces. Thus, imbibition is lost and nutrition of the cartilage is impaired. There is also a decrease in the number of chondrocytes and a loss of proteoglycans.

Grade II: There is a greater degree of cartilage destruction but no exposure of bone. The remaining cartilage is deeper with more loss of chondrocytes and collagen fibers. Grade II is essentially more severe than Grade I.

Grade III: There is a loss of cartilage along with exposure of bony surface. The subchondral bone is exposed.

Grade IV: There is total loss of cartilage along with gross unevenness and remodeling of the bony surface. The opposing portion of the joint now contacts the bone surface with no cushioning and no lubrication.

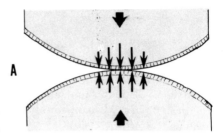

Figure 3–22. Weight distribution on the knee joint: with and without menisci. (A) Without menisci the distribution of weight is concentrated on the center of the contact areas. (B) With menisci weight is distributed along the entire surface of the tibial plateaus and femoral condyles. This explains why every attempt should be made during surgery to salvage any meniscal tissue, and thus minimize degenerative arthritic changes within the cartilage of the femur and tibia. (Modified from Fig. 4–17 in Frankel, VH: Basic Biomechanics of the Skeletal System. Lea & Febiger, Philadelphia, 1980.)

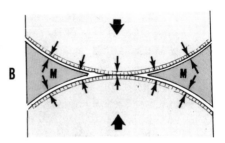

Even though these articular changes are of mechanical origin, as can be deduced by their focal nature (see Fig. 3–22), biochemical changes have been described in these osteoarthritic stages. The gradual loss of proteoglycans causes more water to be imbibed by the cartilage, which impairs physiological nutritive imbibition.[34] The trauma also increases the concentration of lysosomes, which contain proteolytic enzymes that degrade the collagen fiber matrix and cause a gradual loss of elasticity and compressibility

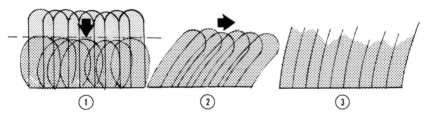

Figure 3–23. Evolution of cartilage degeneration. As shown in Figure 3–22, compression of cartilage causes the collagen "springs" to flatten (*arrow in 1*). Mucin and hyaluronidase are then released to lubricate the joint. This is followed by expansion of the springs, allowing the nutritive fluid to be imbibed.

(2) The lateral translatory force is allowed as long as the collagen fibrils remain intact, but ultimately compression and shear cause the collagen spring to fragment (3), resulting in the loss of compression and elasticity of the collagen.

of the cartilage. The biochemical abnormalities appear to be focal, thus implicating a mechanical origin.

Arthroscopy can be used to visualize cartilage that is structurally and biochemically normal,[35] and this tissue should not be sacrificed. Only abnormally appearing tissue should be excised. The arthroscopist needs to be skilled at distinguishing normal from abnormal menisci.

In summary, what apparently occurs in cartilage breakdown and leads to degenerative arthritis is:

1. A mechanical injury occurs in a localized area as a result of excessive stress or abrasion (shear) (see Fig. 3–22).
2. Proteolytic enzymes are released.
3. The enzymes degrade the matrix.
4. The destruction of the matrix causes a loss of elasticity and impairment of water imbibition.

In addition to, or even possibly instead of, this sequence[36] is the "stiffening" of the subchondral bone, along with microscopic fractures and deformation, which damages the overlying cartilage. These microfractures are allegedly related to repetitive mechanical impulses. Regardless of which theory is correct, the sequence is that of a focal trauma mechanically damaging the cartilage or causing microfractures of the subchondral bone along with proteolytic breakdown and chemical degeneration of the cartilage matrix.

These events are important in proper knee function since the menisci have been estimated to decrease the force exerted on the knee during walking by as much as 3.03 times the body weight.[37] The stress per unit area is 1.6 times greater in the medial compartment than in the lateral compartments and is affected by the menisci.[32]

Healing of damaged cartilage requires a source of chondrocyte cells that can regenerate the matrix, a reasonably intact subchondral plate, and removal or modification of the focus of the mechanical stress, allowing diffuse physiological mechanical stimulation.[38] Since a vascular supply is needed to allow cellular regeneration, salvaging the peripheral area of the meniscus is essential.

CLINICAL MANAGEMENT

Healing of meniscal tears depends on the site, extent, and direction of the tear. Tears that do not extend into the peripheral vascular zone do not heal. Those that do will heal, provided that the displaced remaining meniscus is reduced, preventing further mechanical irritation. Any remaining irregular meniscal tissue that encroaches on the articular cartilage of the femoral condyles or the tibial plateau remains a source of degeneration and, thus, of symptoms.

Conservative (Nonsurgical) Treatment

Conservative management is permissible, and in the opinion of many clinicians desirable, when a specific precise diagnosis is not immediately possible after an acute injury. A more comprehensive examination is possible after the effusion has subsided, quadriceps function has returned, and limited knee function has resumed. The limitation and the reproduction of symptoms during normal daily activities is diagnostic. The purpose of conservative treatment is absorption of the effusion, restoration of quadriceps function, and immediate "unlocking" of the joint.

Reduction of the Locked Knee. The locked knee must be reduced within 24 hours. Allowing the knee to remain locked causes a loss of elasticity of the meniscus; in addition, the meniscus does not return to its normal position within the knee joint.

Removal of effusion is undertaken by immediate application of ice and compression dressings, followed in 48 hours by hot, moist packs. Aspiration under sterile conditions is indicated if the effusion is significant and unremitting. The use of pressure immobilization must be accompanied by simultaneous, isotonic setting quadriceps exercises and should be used for a limited period, not to exceed 3 or 4 days. Oral nonsteroidal anti-inflammatory medications should be initiated, if they are tolerated, to interfere with prostaglandin release.[39]

Manipulation to remove the obstructive aspect of the meniscus tear has been advocated and documented. Manipulation allegedly removes the meniscal fragment from its abnormal site between the femoral condyles and the tibial plateau, and returns it to a region within the knee joint where it can no longer cause mechanical articular damage.[40-42]

The technique of knee manipulation is reasonably simple (Fig. 3–24), but how much force to apply remains problematic since there is the possibility of damage to other tissues, such as ligaments and the joint capsule, as well as further damage to the already impaired meniscus. Manipulation should be skillful, gentle, and without excessive force or "thrust" so that no further injury occurs and the meniscus becomes unlocked.

The technique of reduction by manipulation involves the following steps:

1. Application of longitudinal traction to the lower leg with simultaneous rotation in both directions, and some valgus and varus motion as the knee is being extended.

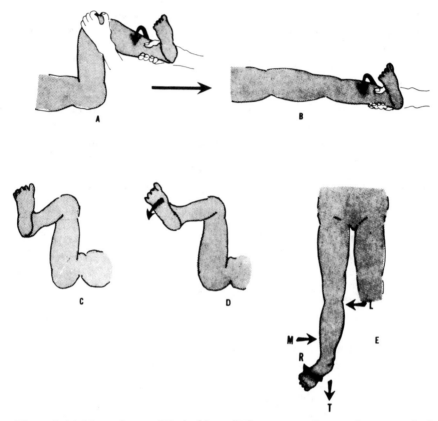

Figure 3–24. Manipulation of "locked knee." The purpose of manipulation to unlock the meniscus is to relieve pain and prevent further damage to the meniscus. (A) In lateral meniscus, the knee is fully flexed and some pressure is exerted to cause varus of the leg (M, medial pressure; L, lateral pressure). (D) The leg is externally rotated. Then the surgeon suddenly (but not forcefully) extends the leg A to B. For lesions of the medial meniscus the opposite motion (internal rotation varus) is used.

    2. If the medial meniscus is suspected as the site of injury, extension is attempted with "internal" rotation being stressed.

    3. If the external meniscus is suspected as the site of injury, external rotation along with extension is stressed. The patient can be requested to forcefully extend ("kick") the knee.

    Once reduced, the full range of active and passive motion in the injured knee must be compared to that of the other knee. Repeated unsuccessful manipulations may cause an extension of the tear into the joint space or indicate that the tear is unreducible and thus reduction must be avoided (Fig. 3–25).

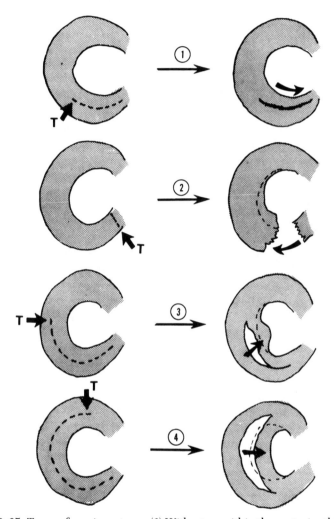

Figure 3–25. Types of meniscus tears. (*1*) With a tear within the posterior third of the meniscus, the elasticity of the cartilage springs the meniscus back into its normal position. (*2*) Posterior tear (T) of the horn's attachment causes the anterior portion to bunch, and locking results. (*3*) A tear (T) halfway to the collateral ligament causes a bunching of the middle portion of the meniscus with similar symptoms to 2. (*4*) If the tear (T) is complete (entire length of the meniscus), the central portion of the meniscus moves toward the center of the joint. This is called a bucket handle tear. No locking occurs because the central fragment is in the intercondylar fossa.

Post Manipulation Reduction. If manipulation has reduced the locking, a rehabilitation program must be immediately started to essentially strengthen the quadriceps and hamstring muscles and to regain and maintain full range of motion. Deep knee bends, squats, and rapid, extensive stair climbing and descending must be avoided. Athletic activities requiring excessive flexion, extension, and rotatory knee action must be avoided.

Frequent and careful examination of the knee must be initiated during the "recovery" phase to ascertain the presence and persistence of meniscal damage and the possibility of additional injury to the collateral and cruciate ligaments. If there is evidence of ligamentous injury resulting from a locked knee, the knee must first be unlocked before the ligamentous injuries are addressed. In the absence of locking, the persistence of effusion may continue for 2 to 3 weeks before a thorough examination is possible. During this period of observation, the state of the quadriceps muscle, as well as range of motion, must be addressed.

In the presence of effusion and even hemarthrosis, an MRI examination is currently the test of choice to fully evaluate the status of the meniscus. Arthrography (Fig. 3–19) is preferably deferred until the effusion subsides.

Surgical Intervention

Treatment originally consisted of nonoperative management or total meniscectomy via arthrostomy. Now, with the advent of arthroscopy, partial meniscectomy and preservation of the remaining normal meniscus is possible.[43] A peripheral tear may, however, require removal of a large portion of the meniscus, thus predisposing the knee to degenerative arthritic changes.[44]

A discussion of surgical technique is beyond the scope of this text and reference is made to the many excellent orthopaedic texts and articles in peer journals of orthopaedics. Long-term follow-up of operated patients is being conducted, and the results are reported in the literature. These studies will ultimately provide better criteria for determining treatment techniques, surgical indications, injury types, and follow-up care. Nevertheless, the competence and experience of the surgeon is still the greatest factor in assuring successful surgical management of the torn meniscus.

Failed surgical treatment, resulting in knee instability, persistent pain, recurrent effusion, joint limitation, and residual functional impairment, may be caused by:

1. Improper or incomplete diagnosis
2. Incompetent and/or inappropriate surgical technique
3. Excessive, prolonged conservative treatment with repeated episodes of locking or "giving way"

4. Pre-existing severe degenerative arthritic changes in the knee, which cause additional meniscal injury

5. Inadequate removal of damaged meniscus, removal of excessive meniscus, or the presence of an overlooked flap

6. Inadequate and/or improper postoperative treatment

7. Premature resumption of traumatic, competitive athletic activities

Postoperative Rehabilitation Program

Immediately postoperatively, even before the tourniquet is removed, the leg should be firmly wrapped in a compressive dressing and elevated. Within the first 24 hours, isometric setting quadriceps exercises should be started. Instruction in these exercises should preferably be initiated prior to the surgery so that the pained postoperative patient is knowledgeable and able to perform the exercises correctly. The importance of these exercises can also be stressed, which will help assure the compliance of the patient. Direct personal instruction is mandatory rather than the mere issuance of a sheet of instructions.

The patient should be instructed to progress gradually from isometric exercise to short-range isotonic exercises. At first the exercises should be performed without resistance; then resistance should be introduced through the inclusion of weights. Since the quadriceps muscle is the main muscle support of the knee joint, a complete discussion of quadriceps exercises is warranted.

Quadriceps Exercises. It has been shown that the entire four muscle bellies of the quadriceps are vital throughout the entire range of knee extension. The concept that the vastus medialis functions exclusively in the last, and most important, range has been refuted. That the quadriceps muscle is of vital importance in knee function has not been questioned.

Exercise, in the broadest sense, can be defined as *purposeful motion.* The muscular, skeletal, and nervous systems are all involved and essentially comprise a single, interdependent system, that is, the neuromusculoskeletal system. Changes are invoked by the performance of exercise. These changes are noted during and immediately after performance of an exercise. There are then adaptive changes that improve function during later episodes of activities demanding exercise. These are termed *training effects* and basically justify the use of exercise as therapy.[45]

Isometric Exercises. Isometric exercises are an accepted type of exercise to ensure that the quadriceps muscle does not atrophy during rest or pain-induced inertia after an acute injury. It is also advocated in the early stage of rehabilitation after injury. The term "isometric" merely implies that the tibiofemoral joint does not move since quadriceps contraction cannot occur without some motion of the patellofemoral joint.

Quadriceps setting can be done in several ways (Fig. 3–26). With the knee fully extended, the quadriceps muscle is slowly and maximally contracted and held for several seconds. This activity is repeated several times each session, and patient should undergo a session hourly. Straight leg raising with the knee extended and a weight attached to the foot-ankle region is a resisted isometric exercise. The resistance can be applied by an elastic cord as shown in Figure 3–26.

Isokinetic Strengthening Exercises. There are several physiological factors to be considered when prescribing exercises, including load, rate, intensity, complexity, coordination, and extent of involvement. The type of stress imposed on the muscle that is to be exercised relates to the function that is to be enhanced. The use of the word "stress" implies that only stress enhances muscular function. Without stress, function cannot be enhanced.

Strength is synonymous with development of tension. Tension is not synonymous with work or power, which involve distance and time factors. Strength can be equated with maximum tension within a muscle produced

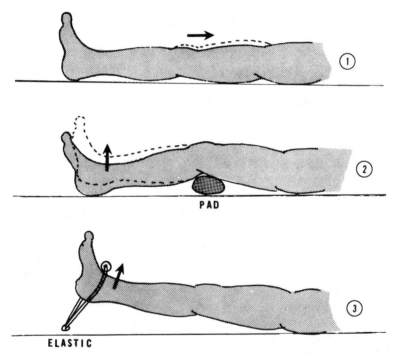

Figure 3–26. Types of quadriceps exercises. (*1*) Setting or isometric exercises with knee fully extended. Joint does not move but muscle shortens: patella moves up. (*2*) Isometric (kinetic) exercise. With a 3-inch-thick pad under the knee, the quadriceps contracts. The joint range of motion is minimal and quadriceps function is enhanced over *1*. (*3*) Increase in exercise with an elastic strap to resist straight leg raising.

by voluntary effort. Certain terms qualify tension, such as "static," which is used when there is no joint movement. A similar term is "isometric contraction." The overall length of the muscle does not change even though there are internal changes within the muscle. The function of isometric contraction is stabilization.

When joint motion accompanies the muscular contraction, the contraction is termed "shortening," "concentric," "isokinetic," or "isotonic." The strength engendered in isotonic contraction is dynamic strength. The use of "iso" is misleading, as it implies equal strength throughout the entire range of motion produced.

The muscle that contracts to resist lengthening undergoes a "lengthening reaction" or "concentric contraction," which is a decelerating force.[46] The maximum tension that is generated during lengthening is significantly greater than that produced during shortening and is considered "negative work."

The number of muscle fibers in a given muscle (in this case, the quadriceps femoris) does not vary significantly from one individual to another but the size of the muscle fibers does. Training influences the size, not the number, and there is evidence that there is an increase in the amount of fibrillar protein.[47]

Strength is increased by recruiting additional motor units rather than by increasing the speed of the firing units. Muscle can therefore literally increase in strength without hypertrophy. Circulatory factors, contrary to many theories, are not important in gaining strength since exercising under arterial occlusion conditions does not reduce maximum tension. Prolonged exercise does deplete available sources of energy and upsets the acid and base balance. Maximum contraction against resistance must be initiated to improve strength.

Endurance implies the ability to continue a specified task over time.[47] Fatigue implies decreased ability of a muscle to generate tension or muscle shortening after a prior activity.

Power, by definition, is the amount of work that can be performed in a finite time, where *work* is defined as the product of force and the distance through which the force is exerted. Power requires that the muscle have a sufficient amount of the correct metabolic ingredients to perform the activity, the ability to replenish these nutrients, and the capability of removing the waste products produced by the contractions. "Conditioning exercises" are now being used as "interval training." Short bursts of high-intensity exercises are followed by equal periods of rest.[48]

DeLorme, a pioneer in exercise physiology, stated, "High force low repetition exercises build strength; low power (force) high repetition builds endurance."[49] This axiom was tested in the excellent study of DeLateur and Lehmann,[46] which considered the transferability of exercise; that is, does one type of exercise ultimately produce the same end result as another type? The study found that there was no transferability between isometric and isotonic exercises.

The results of this study[46] indicate that the true benefit of training was obtained by performing the exercises to the point of fatigue regardless of whether they were low weight or high weight (force). If time and willingness to exercise for a longer period until fatigue are not factors, exercise with intervening periods of rest is more effective, but exercise without a rest period is usually more efficient and does not involve boredom.

How long an exercise program is effective has also been studied. If the individual does not have joint disease or tendonitis, the more exercise, the better. Increases of 12 percent per week have been claimed but vary from 5 to 8 percent, with the greatest degree of improvement in the first 8 weeks.[49]

Equipment. Equipment for the performance of quadriceps exercises varies, and numerous types are currently evolving. The weighted boot (Fig. 3–27) advocated by DeLorme remains popular, economical, and readily available; however, it is cumbersome when an increase in weight is necessary. The essence of *progressive resistance exercise* (PRE) is to determine the maximum resistance that the patient can overcome to fully extend the knee for one contraction (called 1 RM) and to determine the weight that can be lifted to full knee extension for 10 repetitions (10 RM). For the PRE program, the weight of 10 RM is attached to the foot ankle boot, and the knee is extended 10 times and rested for 2 minutes. The weight is slowly lowered. After a full 10 RM repetitions, the knee is maintained at full extension (isometric) with maximum weight for a count of three then slowly lowered (concentric).

This exercise program should take about 30 to 45 minutes and should be done three times a day. Heat applied to the knee before exercise is beneficial and an ice pack afterward relieves any inflammatory reaction.

The resistance (weight of the boot) is increased in increments of 0.5 to 1 lb, and the repetitions are gradually decreased. Gradually a weight that permits only one contraction with maximum effort is reached (1 RM with maximum effort). Once this weight is determined, the exercise is done once three times daily, preceded by heat and followed by ice. Normal power (for that specific individual) is usually reached in 3 to 6 weeks, and a weight of 30 to 35 lbs can be reached by most adults.

The Oxford modification[51] varies from the above DeLorme routine. Here the patient starts with the maximum weight that can be lifted, then does 10 RM with 75 percent maximum weight, then 10 RM with 50 percent weight. Less fatigue occurs. The comparative value remains to be scientifically determined. Both programs are time consuming.

DeLateur and Lehmann[46] advocate finding a weight that the patient can lift three to five times and thereafter count repetitions by metronome until fatigue. The performance is considered a reliable measure of performance.

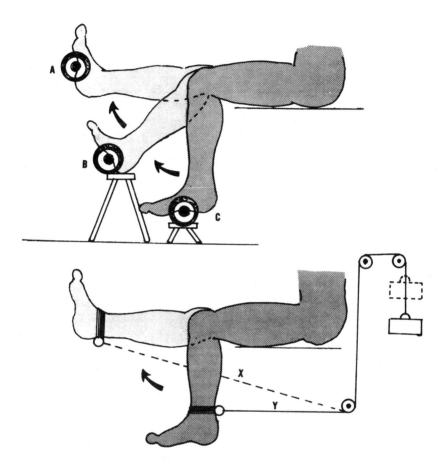

Figure 3–27. Progressive resistive exercises (PRE). (*Top*) The standard technique of PRE with a weighted boot. Full extension is attempted (*A*) and briefly sustained. (*B*) The leg is lowered until the weight and foot are supported to prevent ligamentous stress. *B* causes exercise toward extension from the semiextended position, where the vastus medialis is most effective, rather than from *C*, where resistance against the quadriceps is minimal as the weight pulls vertically along the tibial shaft. In the *C* position there is a greater chance of stress upon the ligaments of the knee from the weighted leg. (*Bottom*) Resistance with pulleys and weights places maximum resistance in the first 45° of extension (*Y*) and decreases as the leg extends, thus placing none (0°) at full extension (*X*).

After a session in which the patient reaches 30 repetitions, the weight is increased and again tried for the initial 3 to 5 repetitions.

Hellebrandt and Houtz[52] advocated keeping the load constant but increasing the rate of contraction. The individual must be able to lift the weight 10 to 20 times at a specific metronome cadence: one contraction per minute. The metronome speed is gradually increased until fatigue is encountered. Endurance as well as strength is attained by this method.

The N-K table (Fig. 3–28) has been developed. The angle between the lever arm and the load arm as well as the weight in this table is more manageable. The Elgin table (Fig. 3–29) involves the hip as well as the knee extensors. Cybex extremity testing and Nautilus equipment are also advocated, but they are expensive and not readily available. In addition, trained personnel are needed to monitor their use. All these pieces of equipment are available as well as literature that proclaim their virtues.

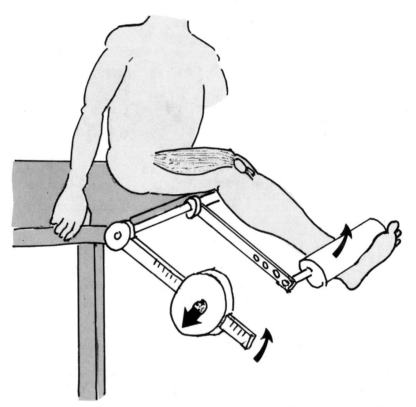

Figure 3–28. Quadriceps exercise equipment: N-K table. The N-K table, available in many physical therapy departments, is more efficient than the boot because the weight can be adjusted merely by sliding it up and down. The angle can also change the resistance, which is not uniform throughout the entire range of extension.

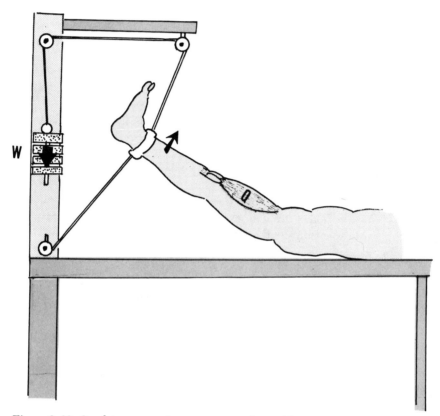

Figure 3–29. Quadriceps exercise equipment: Elgin table. With the patient supine, the extended leg is lifted against resistance that is graded by changing the weights (W). The exercise can be done isometrically and isokinetically and in acceleration and deceleration. This exercise does not strengthen the quadriceps (Q) throughout its flexion-extension range of motion. There are cams and pulleys within the equipment that direct the resistance.

It is apparent that the ideal method of quadriceps exercise has not been developed or, at least, universally accepted. Maximum contraction and endurance must be achieved through a daily program, and isotonic as well as isometric strength must be acquired. Concentric contraction, the slow release of contraction, must also be performed.

Hamstring Strengthening Exercise. In treating knee problems, the strength and flexibility of the hamstring muscle group are often overlooked. The isokinetic strength of the hamstring is not used in everyday activities, but the hamstring muscle must have sufficient flexibility to not obstruct or impair quadriceps contraction strength and range. The hamstrings also decelerate the leg in ambulation and in athletic activities. A stretching and strengthening program (Fig. 3–30) must be undertaken in all patients with knee problems.

Exercises to Strengthen Ligaments. Ligaments have been shown to increase their tensile strength from progressive gentle stretching (Fig. 3–31). Even partial tears as well as ligamentous stretch injuries to ligaments respond well to gentle progressive active stretching. As ligaments are so vital in the stability of the femorotibial knee joint, it is necessary that ligaments as well as the muscles of the knee be strengthened. Ligaments are beneficially involved in the active muscle exercises given, but additional passive stretching exercises address the ligaments more specifically in a rehabilitation program.

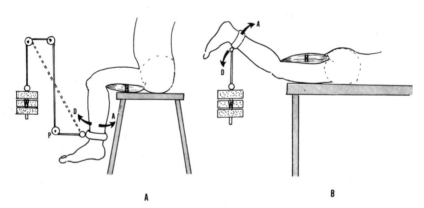

A   B

Figure 3–30. Hamstring exercises. (A) The seated patient is exercising the hamstring muscle (H) against a weight (W). Isokinetic acceleration (A) and deceleration (D) are depicted. The pulley (P) can be changed (*as shown by the dotted line*) so that the range of muscle contraction and elongation can be varied. (B) A similar hamstring exercise in the prone position against resistance (W) is shown. Again acceleration (A) and deceleration (D) are depicted.

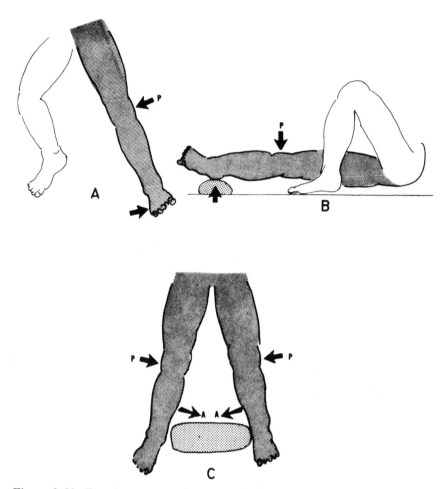

Figure 3–31. Exercises to stress ligaments of the knee. Both medial and lateral collateral ligaments are stretched daily as part of the exercise program on the assumption that gentle but firm and repeated stress upon the ligaments increases their resilience. *A* and *B* indicate how the patient stretches manually the medial ligament. (*C*) With the use of a firm pillow both active (A) and passive (P) exercises stretch and stress the ligaments. Exercises weighted against gravity also stress and strengthen ligaments.

REFERENCES

1. Goldman, A and Waugh, TR: Menisci of the knee: A review paper. Orthop Review 14(2):67, 1985.
2. Cailliet, R. In Sidney Licht, (ed): Mechanics of Joints: Arthritis and Physical Medicine. Elizabeth Licht Publisher, New Haven, 1969, p 17.
3. Frankel, VH, Burstein, AB, and Brooks, DB: Biomechanics of internal derangements of the knee. J Bone Joint Surg 53A:945, 1971.
4. Galeazzi, R: Clinical and experimental study of lesions of the semilunar cartilage of the knee joint. Journal Bone Joint Surg 9:515, 1927.
5. Kaplan, EB: The lateral meniscofemoral ligaments of the knee joint. Bull Hosp Joint Dis 17:176, 1956.
6. Basmajian, JV and Lovejoy, JF: Functions of the popliteus muscle in man. J Bone Joint Surg 53A:557, 1971.
7. Bullough, PGA, et al: The strength of the menisci of the knee as it relates to their fine structure. J Bone Joint Surg 32B:564, 1970.
8. King, DK: The healing of semilunar cartilage. J Bone Joint Surg 18:1069, 1936.
9. MacConnaill, MA: The function of intraarticular fibrocartilages with special reference to the knee and inferior radioulnar joints. J Anat 64:210, 1932.
10. Swann, DA, et al: Role of hyaluronic acid in joint lubrication. Ann Rheum Dis 33:318, 1974.
11. Fairbank, TJ: Knee joint changes after meniscectomy. J Bone Joint Surg 30B:664, 1948.
12. Kettlekamp, DB and Jacobs, AW: Tibiofemoral contact area: Determination and implications. J Bone Joint Surg 54A:349, 1972.
13. Cailliet, R: The walking foot. In Cailliet, R (ed): Foot and Ankle Pain. FA Davis, Philadelphia, 1968, p 45.
14. Krause, WR, et al: Mechanical changes in the knee after meniscectomy. J Bone Joint Surg 64A:600, 1982.
15. Voto, SJ and Ewing, A: Nomenclature system for meniscal lesions of the knee. Surg Rounds Orthop 34, 1989.
16. Sprague, NF: Arthroscopic surgery: Degenerative and traumatic flap tears of the meniscus. Contemp Orthop 9(4):23, 1964.
17. Dandy, DJ: The arthroscopic anatomy of symptomatic meniscal lesions. J Bone Joint Surg 72B(4):628, 1990.
18. DeHaven, KE: Diagnosis of acute knee injuries with hemarthrosis. Am J Sports Med 8(1):9, 1980.
19. O'Donoghue, DH: Surgical treatment of fresh injuries to the major ligaments of the knee. J Bone Joint Surg 31A:721, 1950.
20. Jackson, RW and DeHaven, KE: Arthroscopy of the knee. Clin Orthop 107:87, 1975.
21. de Andrade, JR, Grant, C, and St J. Dixon, A: Joint distension and reflex muscle inhibition in the knee. J Bone Joint Surg 47A(2):313, 1965.
22. Lieb, FJ and Perry, J: Quadriceps function: An anatomical and mechanical study using amputated limbs. J Bone Joint Surg 50A:1535, 1968.
23. Mink, J: Magnetic Resonance Investigation of the Musculoskeletal System. Raven Press, 1990.
24. Noble, J and Erat, K: In defence of the meniscus: A prospective study of 200 meniscectomy patients. J Bone Joint Surg 62B(1):7, 1980.
25. Watson-Jones, R: Fractures and Joint Injuries. E & S Livingstone Ltd., Edinburgh, 1956, p 769.
26. Johnson, RJ, et al: Factors affecting late results after meniscectomy. J Bone Joint Surg 56A:719, 1974.
27. Gear, MWL: The late results of meniscectomy. Br J Surg 54:270, 1967.

28. Appel, H: Late results after meniscectomy in the knee joint. Acta Orthop Scand (Suppl.): 133, 1970.
29. Lipscomb, PR and Henderson, MS: Internal derangements of the knee. JAMA 135:827, 1947.
30. Editorial: Unnecessary meniscectomy. Lancet 1:235, 1976.
31. Dandy, DJ and Jackson, RW: The impact of arthroscopy on the management of disorders of the knee. J Bone Joint Surg, 1975, p 346.
32. Rand, JA: Arthroscopy and articular cartilage defects. Contemp Orthop 11(4):13, 1985.
33. Cailliet, R: Arthritis and physical medicine. In Sidney Licht (ed): Mechanics of Joints. Waverly Press, Baltimore, 1969, p 17.
34. Mankin, HJ: The reaction of articular cartilage to injury and osteoarthritis. N Engl J Med 291:1335, 1974.
35. Brockhurst, R, et al: The composition of normal and osteoarthritic articular cartilage from human knee joints. J Bone Joint Surg 64A(1):95, 1984.
36. Radin, EL: The physiology and degeneration of joints. Semin Arthritis Rheum 2(3):245, 1972–1973.
37. Morrison, JB: The mechanics of the knee joint in relation to normal walking. J Biomechanics 3:51, 1970.
38. Mankin, HJ: Current concepts review: The response of articular cartilage to mechanical injury. J Bone Joint Surg 64A:460, 1982.
39. Chrisman, OD, Ladenbauer-Bellis, IM, Panjabi, M, and Goeltz, S: The relationship of mechanical trauma and early biochemical reactions of osteoarthritic cartilage. Clin Orthop 161:275, 1981.
40. Cyriax, J: Textbook of Orthopedic Medicine, Vol 2: Treatment by Manipulation, Massage and Injection. Williams & Wilkins, Baltimore, 1971, p 366.
41. Paterson, JK and Bum, L: An Introduction to Medical Manipulation. MTP Press Limited, Boston, 1985, p 127.
42. Maitland, GD: Peripheral Manipulation, ed 2. Butterworths, London, 1979, p 230.
43. Hanks, GA and Kalenak, A: Alternative arthroscopic techniques for meniscal repair: A review. Orthop Review 19(6):541, 1990.
44. Jackson, JP: Degenerative changes in the knee after meniscectomy. Br Med J 2:525, 1968.
45. Darling, RC: Exercise. In Downey, JA and Darling, RC (eds): Physiological Basis of Rehabilitation Medicine. WB Saunders, Philadelphia, 1971, p 167.
46. DeLateur, BJ and Lehmann, JF: Therapeutic exercise to develop strength and endurance. In Kottke, FJ and Lehmann, FL (eds): Krusen's Handbook of Physical Medicine and Rehabilitation. WB Saunders, Philadelphia, 1990, p 480.
47. Barnard, RJ, Edgerton, VR, and Peter, JB: Effect of exercise on skeletal muscle. I. Biochemical and histochemical properties. J Appl Physiol 28:762, 1970.
48. Astrand, I, et al: Intermittent muscular work. Acta Physiol Scand 48:448, 1960.
49. DeLorme, TL: Restoration of muscle power by heavy-resistance exercises. J Bone Joint Surg 27A:645, 1945.
50. Ko, I: Training of muscle strength and power: Interaction of neuromotoric, hypertrophic and mechanical factors. Int J Sports Med 7(Suppl.):10, 1986.
51. Zinovieff, AN: Heavy resistance exercises: The "Oxford" technique. Br J Phys Med 14:129, 1967.
52. Hellebrandt, FA and Houtz, SJ. Methods of muscle training: The influence of pacing. Phys Therap Rev 38:319, 1958.

CHAPTER 4

Ligamentous Injuries

It can be assumed from a review of structural and functional anatomy, discussed in Chapters 1 and 2, that knee stability relies primarily on ligamentous structure. This is true of both the static and the kinetic knee.

The incongruity of the articular surfaces comprising the knee joint, the femoral condyles and the tibial plateau, demand the intrusion of the menisci and the integrity of the collateral and cruciate ligaments. The muscles and their tendons are involved only slightly in stability, but they function primarily in motion and reinforcment of the ligaments when they fail or are overwhelmed. The structure of the joint capsule does not provide sufficient support or stability.

The structure of the ligaments involves their component collagen fibers and their alignment. Ligaments are composed of structurally parallel collagen fibers that attach to the periosteum of the opposing joint cartilaginous surfaces. Their function is to limit movement considered as being within physiological range. The normal elasticity of collagen is the limit to which the trihelical peptide chain uncoils (Fig. 4–1).[1]

The elongation of ligament collagen fibers can be exceeded by (1) internal disruption, (2) separation of their terminal portion from their periosteal attachment, or (3) avulsion of a small fraction of the bone to which the tendon is attached. In analyzing internal disruption, the collagen fibers can be partially elongated with some fibers remaining intact or the fibers can be completely severed, which causes total disruption. The former is a stretched fiber and the latter is a torn fiber.

The cruciate ligaments have a different arrangement of collagen fibers that is functionally pertinent to the elasticity of that ligament (Fig. 4–2).

Excessive joint motion, that is, exceeding the physiological joint range of motion, occurs essentially at the expense of ligamentous resistance. When such a joint is exposed to trauma, it is considered to be "subluxed" or

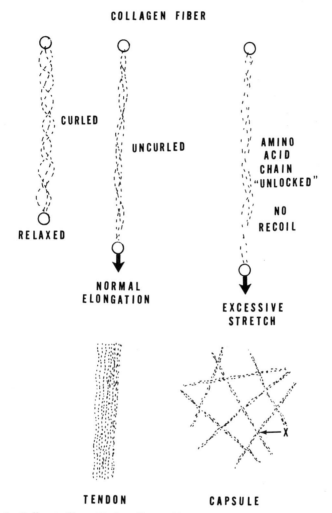

COLLAGEN FIBER

CURLED

RELAXED

UNCURLED

NORMAL
ELONGATION

AMINO
ACID
CHAIN
"UNLOCKED"

NO
RECOIL

EXCESSIVE
STRETCH

TENDON   CAPSULE

Figure 4–1. Collagen fiber. Each collagen fiber is a trihelical chain of amino acids bound together chemically. They uncurl to their physiologic length, then recoil when the elongation force is released. If the collagen fiber is elongated past its physiologic length, the amino acid chains become disrupted and the fiber no longer returns to its resting length.

A tendon consists of parallel bands of collagen fibers. In a capsule, the collagen fibers crisscross and glide over each other at their intersection (X). The capsule depicted here elongates as far as each collagen fiber permits.

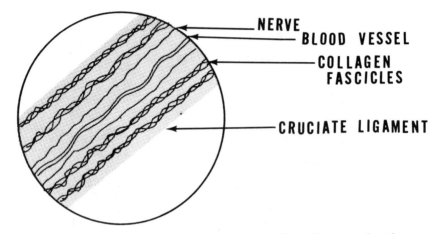

NERVE

BLOOD VESSEL

COLLAGEN
FASCICLES

CRUCIATE LIGAMENT

Figure 4–2. Microscopic view of cruciate ligament. The collagenous fascicles are undulated in a slight manner, allowing little elongation. The blood vessels are tortuous but again slight. There are nerves within the ligament that subserve pain sensation. The structure explains the limited elasticity of the cruciate ligament.

"luxed," depending on the severity of the stressing injury and the joint response to that trauma.

The term "luxation" is applied to displacement of articular surfaces, that is, dislocation of a joint.[2] The term "subluxation" refers to a lesser degree of luxation in which the joint surfaces have changed in their relationship but, to a degree, remain associated as compared to total luxation in which the articular surfaces are totally dissociated.

Terms that have been applied to these mechanical subluxations include strain and sprain. Strain means "to injure by making too strong an effort or by excessive use."[2] In this concept, it is a verb denoting an action on a tissue: in this case the tendon reaction from the subluxing or luxing of a joint. Sprain, from the French "espraindre" implies "trauma to a joint that causes pain and disability depending upon degree of injury to ligaments. In severe sprain, ligaments may be completely torn."[2]

These are dictionary definitions of the words, whereas, clinically, the differentiation of strain versus sprain has specific diagnostic and therapeutic implications. Excessive joint motion that results in a ligamentous injury constitutes a sprain. The insult, with resultant joint reaction, is the strain. Thus, *strain* may be considered to be the physical force imposed on the ligamentous tissues, conceivably exceeding normal resiliency but not, per se, causing or resulting in residual deformation or damage to the tissues. Physiological recovery may be anticipated in mere strain. *Sprain*, semantically, is the tissue reaction to strain with resultant deformation or damage to the (joint) tissues. Expected recovery, here, will depend on the extent of structural deformation, the incurred structural damage and the ensuing treatment.

A knee injury that is considered a strain and the possible resultant sprain needs to be evaluated to determine:

1. The precise force imposed
2. The precise position of the knee at the moment of impact
3. The direction of the force
4. The guarding muscular action effective at the moment of the impact, which could dispel or decrease the significance of the impact
5. The pre-existing condition of the affected tissues

Force analysis determines which tissue (ligament or meniscus) may be involved. The determination of the force indicates the possible degree of sprain reaction. If a ligament injury is suspected, the diagnostic challenge is to determine which ligament and what degree of injury has occurred. Meniscal injury is considered in another chapter, but suffice it to say at this point, several types of tissue may be injured during a single incident and the examiner cannot be lulled into assuming that only one tissue is involved as a result of a specific injury. It must also be stated that several ligaments, as well as other tissues, may be injured.

The clinical evidence required for determining the precise ligament that has been injured mandates that normal anatomical structures and the result of laboratory division of separate ligaments be known. A determination must be made of abnormal joint movement after precise division of the knee ligaments has occurred.[3] The functional aspects of each ligament must be ascertained, and the resultant knee instability therefore appreciated in a meaningful clinical examination. It must be recognized that it would literally be impossible to sustain a complete tearing of one ligament without some damage to other structures in the knee joint.

PATHOLOGICAL ANATOMY

From the history, the precise position of the knee can be determined and the direction of force on the ligamentous structures can be ascertained. This information can indicate to the examiner which ligament(s) is involved. Classic tests have, over the years, been established without an accurate anatomical knowledge. These tests have frequently given inaccurate information. Fresh cadaver studies have elicited the precise abnormal movement that results from division of one or a combination of knee ligaments.[3]

In the completely extended knee both collateral and cruciate ligaments are taut. In this position the condyles of the femur and the tibial plateau are congruous (fit closely), giving anatomical stability. As "full knee extension" varies in different individuals, normal extension for that patient must be determined through examination of the contralateral side.

Immediately on incurring a degree of flexion, some degree of rotation becomes possible because the ligaments become relaxed. The collateral ligaments relax, and the cruciate ligament remains taut, albeit to a lesser degree. Normally, continued flexion of the knee includes internal rotation (see Chap. 2). Rotation varies from 5° to 20°, with more external rotation than internal rotation.

The axis of normal rotation is not central. In rotation the lateral tibial condyle rotates predominantly, causing the axis to migrate medially with no subluxation normally occurring. When the ligaments are divided, subluxation of the condyles can result, causing a shift of the axis.

The medial ligament has three portions: the superficial, deep, and oblique portions. The superficial portion is vertical, descending slightly forward in the extended knee. As the knee flexes, the superficial layer glides on the deep layer, which is a thick, strong structure derived from the joint capsule. The peripheral edge of the meniscus is attached to this deep ligament.

Abnormal motion that occurs after division of the *medial collateral ligament* (MCL) depends on the level of the division. Division of the ligament at the bony attachment to the tibia does not result in abnormal motion in full knee extension, but with only a few degrees of flexion abnormal rotation results, increasing as flexion proceeds to 90°. Increasing flexion causes the medial tibial condyle to rotate externally and produces marked forward subluxation of the condyle. At this point the posterior horn of the meniscus restricts further abnormal rotation (the "door stop" effect). Further rotation occurs if the meniscus is removed. This meniscus action is probably the reason that this portion of the meniscus may tear as a result of a ligamentous injury.

Excessive rotation places the anterior cruciate ligament at an angle over the lateral femoral condyle, which then may tear (ligament). This is another example of an initial medial collateral ligamentous tear that may, if excessive, lead to a tear of the meniscus and ultimately to a tear of the *anterior cruciate ligament* (ACL).

The direction of the anterior cruciate ligament reveals the control it exerts in preventing abnormal motion of the knee joint. It extends forward and medially from the rear aspect of the lateral femoral condyle to the front of the intercondylar area of the tibia. As previously stated, the ACL is taut in full knee extension and flexion as well as in midflexion when the knee is internally rotated, a physiological state (Fig. 4–3). The ACL is only slightly relaxed in external rotation of the tibia on the femur.

The fact that the ACL is taut at full extension, full flexion, and midflexion with internal rotation indicates why a force imposed on the knee in these positions can possibly cause a tear. As will be seen in the discussion

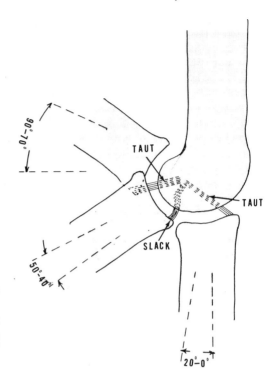

Figure 4–3. Anterior cruciate ligament during knee flexion. The anterior cruciate ligament is taut at full (0°) flexion, then again becomes taut at 70° to 80° flexion.

of knee tests, these observations negate the diagnostic specificity of the flexed knee (90°) drawer test for ACL instability and brings into question the advisability of testing at 5° to 15° of flexion.[4] It becomes apparent also that abnormal motion is not merely *anterior subluxation* but anterior subluxation of the lateral tibial tubercle, resulting in *anterolateral instability*.

Division of the MCL and ACL does not affect stability at full knee extension, but there is demonstrable instability immediately on slight flexion. Thus the method of performing the standard *valgus stress test* must be analyzed. Performance of the valgus stress test with the knee fully extended can now be seen to be invalid since the medial aspect of the knee joint does not significantly open until a few degrees of flexion has been produced. Even in the presence of a torn *posterior cruciate ligament* (PCL) and a torn medial collateral ligament, there is a negative valgus stress test. The medial joint space opens significantly only when there is division of the medial collateral ligaments and both cruciate ligaments. It does open palpably when the superficial ligament is torn.

Admittedly, injury to the cruciate ligaments has been considered the injury with the greatest potential for significant to severe functional impairment. However, injury to the collateral ligaments also occurs in today's contact sports and vehicular accidents.

Today, many medical authors favor primary surgical repair for complete rupture of collateral ligaments of the knee. Nevertheless, reports of nonsurgical care of tears of the medial collateral ligament appear more frequently in the medical literature. The key to the initiation of successful appropriate nonsurgical treatment appears to be establishing that the cruciate ligaments are intact.

The functional anatomy of the MCL has been discussed in Chapter 2, but a brief review is indicated to substantiate appropriate diagnosis and resultant conservative treatment. As stated, the MCL is complex and multilayered. It originates from the medial femoral condyle and crosses the knee joint in a slight posterior to anterior direction to insert on the medial region of the tibia under the anterior border of the pes anserinus muscle. It is superficial to the deeper capsular ligamentous complex, so it has been labeled the "superficial medial collateral ligament." Posteriorly the superficial layer blends with the posterior medial capsule of the deeper portion, forming what is termed the "posterior oblique ligament" of the knee.

The function of the MCL is to limit the opening of the joint when a valgus force is applied to the knee. The anterior portion of the MCL performs most of this function. After section of the MCL, only 3 to 5 mm of joint separation occurs.[5] Prior to complete failure of the MCL, the deeper medial capsular structures must also fail.[6] These findings indicate that nonsurgical repair of the MCL must be predicated on the intactness of the deep capsular portion.

MEDIAL COLLATERAL LIGAMENT

The vast majority of MCL injuries are the result of severe valgus forces applied to the inner aspect of the knee and usually with the knee slightly flexed at the moment of impact. The impact may be the result of a vehicular or athletic accident.

Signs and Symptoms

Usually little or no pain is experienced immediately after the injury. More commonly the complaint is "weakness" rather than pain. Tenderness over the medial aspect of the knee is experienced or produced by the examiner.

Examination must be properly and accurately performed.[7] The patient must be completely relaxed and the quadriceps flaccid. Essentially the patella must be able to move freely and the quadriceps should be totally relaxed. The examiner flexes the knee slightly, which relaxes the posterior portion of the capsular ligament, and places the tibia in an externally rotated position. This position prevents any possible rotation during the examination, which could falsify its interpretation. The extended valgus force by the examiner must be gentle.

The testing determines the degree of opening as compared to that of the contralateral knee, which is then similarly examined. The quality of the *end point feel* is important and requires experience on the part of the examiner. In the normal knee there is a distinct end point that is missing in the injured one. All traditional cruciate signs, Lachman, Losee, drawer signs, and pivot shift, must be negative.

Treatment Protocol

The treatment protocol of Indelicato[7] has three phases.

Phase 1. Immediately after diagnosis the knee is placed in a prefabricated orthosis that holds the knee at 30° of flexion. Isometric quadriceps exercises (described in Chap. 3) are initiated immediately and are done several times daily with gradual resistance. Partial weight bearing may be instituted. Isokinetic quadriceps exercises of the other leg against resistance are indicated in the anticipation that there will be crossover benefit for the injured knee.

Phase 2. Phase 2 begins after the second week and continues until the sixth week. A hinge that permits knee motion from 30° to 90° is placed on the orthosis. Full extension is prevented. Isokinetic quadriceps exercises (described in Chap. 3) are begun between these ranges and with increasing resistance. Full weight-bearing ambulation is permitted.

Phase 3. Phase 3 begins at the sixth week. The orthosis is completely removed. Isokinetic exercises are continued with increasing resistance and frequency to regain strength, power, and endurance (see Chap. 3). When testing reveals that 60 percent of strength has been regained, running may be added to ambulation, and exercise is continued until 80 percent of strength is regained. Full athletic activities are permitted without a knee brace.

Other authors[8] have different protocols, but it is possible that their patients had other impairments, such as ACL or meniscal damage. If there is a question of other injuries, an arthroscopic examination may be performed to confirm or refute the presence of other pathologies. Effusion or hemarthrosis may imply additional damage.

The lateral aspect of the knee is protected by four structures:

1. The lateral collateral ligaments
2. The fascia lata
3. The popliteus tendon
4. The biceps femoris

An injury of sufficient force to tear the lateral support structures must involve all four to cause instability.

The lateral collateral ligament is taut in full knee extension and very relaxed in full flexion. In rotation the ligament becomes tight but not taut, as has been shown in autopsy studies in which complete isolated division of the lateral collateral ligament causes minimal change in stability. Extreme external rotation is resisted by the ACL, and abnormal external rotation is limited by the two cruciate ligaments and the MCL.

Varus strain on the extended knee does not open the joint space and even with knee flexion, it opens very little. Division of the lateral ligament with division of either cruciate ligament will not open the joint space with the knee fully extended. It will open widely with the knee flexed, but only when both cruciates are severed will it open in full knee extension.

Posterior cruciate ligament division allows a positive posterior drawer test from 10° of flexion and is at a maximum at 90° of flexion. There is a negative posterior drawer test with the knee fully extended.

Division of the posterior cruciate together with severance of the collateral ligament results in posterior subluxation of the tibia, especially of the lateral tibial condyle. Division of the posterior cruciate together with severance of the medial collateral ligament results in posterior subluxation of the tibia and gross abnormality of both anterior and posterior rotation of the medial tibial condyles.

LATERAL LIGAMENTOUS INJURY

The anatomy of the lateral collateral ligament has been fully discussed in Chapters 1 and 2 and will not be repeated here.

Injury to the lateral ligaments of the knee occurs less often than does injury to the ACL or MCL but has potentially severe sequelae. Injury to this ligament occurs primarily from athletic activity or violent motor vehicle accidents. Lateral ligament injuries often result from knee dislocations[9,10] and may have a residual peroneal nerve palsy.[11] The severity of the sequelae emphasize the need for the recognition and treatment of this injury.

Most, if not all, lateral collateral ligamentous tears involve injury of the fibular collateral ligament, as well as the arcuate ligament, the biceps tendon, and the iliotibial band.

Examination reveals excessive varus, 5 mm or more of opening, when the varus stress is applied (Fig. 4–4). The varus test is utilized for diagnosis of cruciate ligament injuries but initially also indicates that the lateral collateral ligament tears first, causing excessive opening of the lateral joint space. X-rays often reveal avulsion fractures of the fibula and indicate lateral capsular tears. In addition, x-rays reveal the extent of lateral joint space

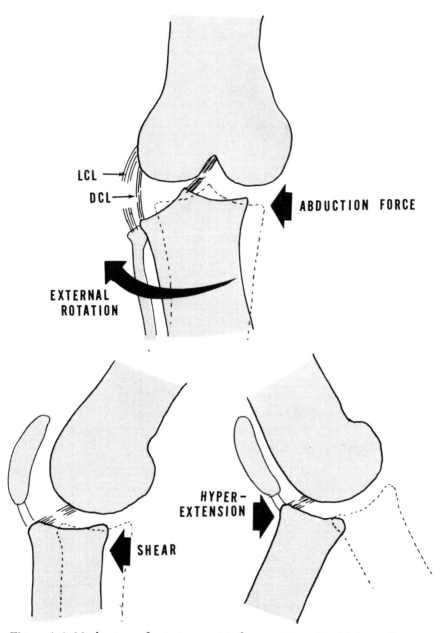

Figure 4–4. Mechanisms of anterior cruciate ligament tear. (*Top*) Injury of severe external rotation with abduction injury. The lateral collateral ligament (LCL) tears first, then the deep capsular ligament (DCL), last is the tear of the anterior cruciate ligament. Anterior shear and severe hyperextension of the knee can also tear the anterior cruciate ligament.

opening on varus stressing. Arthroscopy may ultimately be more diagnostically accurate, but there are few reports of its use.

Specific treatment of lateral collateral ligamentous tears, either operative or nonoperative conservative treatment, is not currently agreed on
universally.

ANTERIOR CRUCIATE LIGAMENT
DISRUPTION

The anatomical structure of the anterior cruciate ligament is described
in Chapter 1 and its function in Chapter 2. The ACL is the major stabilizer
of the knee and thus plays an increasingly important role in clinical
orthopedics.

ACL disruption was first described by Stark in 1850[12] and has today
become a significant disabling condition of the knee. This is a frequent
athletic injury and is one of the most disabling types. It is a major cause of
interruption of athletic careers.

The clinical diagnosis of a suspect anterior cruciate ligament disruption
was initially determined by eliciting a positive drawer sign (Fig. 4–5). This

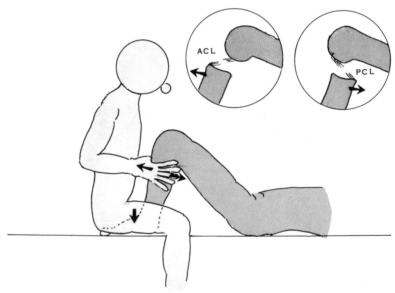

Figure 4–5. Drawer sign test for cruciate ligaments. The standard drawer sign test for
cruciate ligaments immobilizes the foot and stresses the lower leg on the femur.
Pulling the leg forward tests the anterior cruciate ligament (ACL) and posterior
pressure tests the posterior cruciate ligament (PCL).

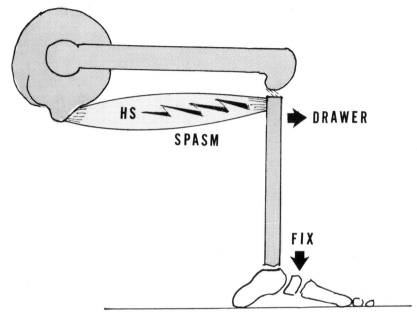

Figure 4–6. False negative drawer sign due to hamstring spasm. In spite of torn or elongated ACL, the drawer sign test may be negative because the torn ACL induces a protective spasm in the hamstring muscles. The fact that the tibia cannot be pulled forward in the test implies an adequate ACL when it is really held there by the hamstring spasm.

test reveals excessive translation of the tibia on the femur when the knee is flexed at 90°. Excessive translation indicates that the restrictive action of the ACL is impaired. The examiner, holding the foot firmly on the examining table, applies force on the tibia in an anterior direction. The degree of translation is compared to that of the contralateral knee.

False negative results for the drawer sign test are attributed to the following:

1. The usual hemarthrosis resulting from tearing of the ACL precludes flexing of the knee to a full 90° as well as the tensing of the entire knee joint capsule.

2. A protective "spasm" of the hamstring muscles in the well-muscled athlete negates any significant anterior translation (Fig. 4–6).

3. Anatomically the concavities of the two articulating joint surfaces inhibit translation at 90° of knee flexion (Fig. 4–7). The posterior aspect of the femoral condyles is acutely convex as compared to the opposing articular surface of the tibia, which is level. The medial meniscus moves with the tibia so that in performing the translation of the tibia on the femur, the posterior

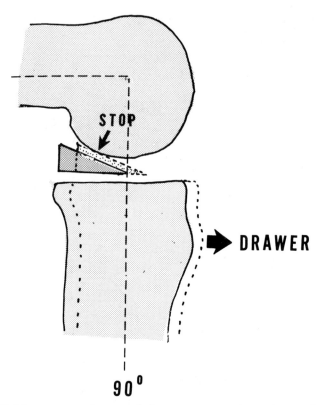

Figure 4–7. Meniscus interfering with drawer sign test. Since the standard drawer sign test has the knee flexed at 90°, the meniscus can act as a door stop, thus preventing the tibia from moving forward. It is thus impossible to judge an ACL abnormality. The stopping of forward movement implies an adequate ACL, whereas when the forward movement is stopped by the meniscus, the ACL may be torn or elongated.

width of the meniscus acts like a door stop, mechanically preventing further anterior translation.

A positive anterior drawer sign test can only occur if there is a significant loss of the posterior horn of the meniscus, disruption of the medial capsular ligament, or disruption of the posterior oblique ligaments, allowing separation of the condyles with the tibial plateau. Merely having a tear of the ACL is not sufficient to produce a positive test.

Lachman Test

A more specific diagnostic sign was proposed in 1976 by Lachman (quoted in Gurtier et al.[13]), which has subsequently been accepted as being reliable as well as accurate. The test is performed by:

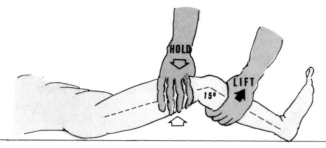

Figure 4–8. Technique for performing the Lachman maneuver in testing the adequacy of the anterior cruciate ligament. With the patient supine and the involved leg facing the examiner, the thigh is firmly grasped above the knee (hold) and the tibia is grasped below the knee (lift). The leg is held extended or flexed not more than 15°.

While holding the thigh, the tibia is pulled upward, and the distance it moves against the femur is compared to the other normal knee. The ACL normally restricts this motion. When the ACL is torn or elongated, the tibia moves excessively against the femoral condyles.

1. Having the patient lie supine on the table with the involved leg next to the examiner.

2. Holding the patient's knee between full extension and 15° of flexion.

3. Stabilizing the femur with one hand while applying firm upward pressure against the posterior aspect of the proximal tibia with the other hand, attempting anterior translation of the tibia (Fig. 4–8).

The meniscus does not intervene in this test since it is done with the leg fully extended or flexed no more than 15°. The configuration of the anterior portion of the femoral condyles and the more horizontal plane of the tibial plateau do not permit the door stop effect (Fig. 4–9) as observed in the 90° flexed drawer test. The angle of the tibia during the Lachman test also

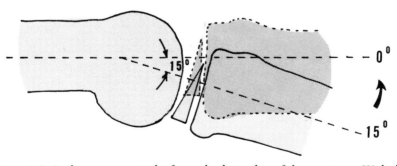

Figure 4–9. Lachman concept: tibiofemoral relationship of the meniscus. With the knee extending from 15° flexion to full extension (0°), the meniscus does not act as a door stop, giving a false negative ACL sign.

eliminates, or at least diminishes, the possibility that a hamstring spasm could give a false negative test.

A positive Lachman test, indicating disruption of the ACL, is considered when there is a "mushy" end point to anterior translation of the tibia, and the translation on the affected side is greater than on the normal side. In the presence of an intact ACL, there is a firm (hard) end point of anterior tibial translation.

The position of the examiner's hands is important. One hand must firmly immobilize the femur and the hand on the tibia must be placed so that the thumb lies on the anterior medial margin of the knee joint. In this position the exact degree of anterior translation movement at the joint can be palpated by the thumb (Fig. 4–10).

The classical Lachman test is performed by having the patient lie supine while the examiner holds the thigh with one hand. Today many athletes are so muscular, with massive thigh girth, that it is difficult if not impossible for the average examiner to firmly hold the thigh with one hand. Since the goal of the test is the "end feel" of the tibial translation an ingenious variation of the Lachman test has been described[14] that facilitates doing the test. It can essentially be termed the *reversed Lachman test* and employs the following basic principles (Fig. 4–11):

1. The patient lies prone with the involved leg on the same side of the table as the examiner.

2. The knee is held in a flexed position (15° to 30° of flexion) by placing the examiner's knee under the ankle.

3. Two fingers can palpate the anterior point margin to ascertain the end point of movement. The other examining hand presses downward and

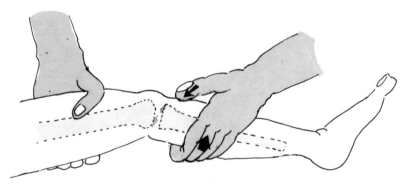

Figure 4–10. Position of thumb in the Lachman test. The hand that is on the tibia and elevates it (*large arrow*) should have its thumb (*small arrow*) placed upon the anterior aspect of the tibia below the patella to appreciate any subluxation of the tibia upon the femur (in case of inadequacy of the ACL).

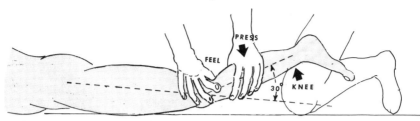

Figure 4–11. Reversed Lachman test for ACL inadequacy. In a very muscular large person the standard Lachman test may be difficult since the average examiner's hand cannot stabilize the thigh. With the patient prone, the examiner can place a knee under the lower leg just above the ankle and place the knee at 30° of flexion. With downward pressure (press) upon the upper calf, excessive anterior translation of the tibia can be felt (feel) by the examiner's other hand that is palpating the tibiofemoral joint space. A positive Lachman test can be ascertained by a comparison with the other normal leg.

forward on the upper calf. A mushy resistance rather than a firm end point can be determined.

In this position, the posterior cruciate ligament can also be evaluated by lifting the lower leg. The posterior drawer test is done in the prone position.

The Lachman test is graded in the following manner:

Grade I. There is a feeling of a soft, mushy end point in anterior translation of the tibia as compared to a hard end point. This is termed *proprioceptive appreciation* and is considered a positive Lachman sign.

Grade II. There is visible as well as palpable excessive anterior translation of the tibia. This is seen by looking laterally at the knee joint during the test. The normal slope of the infrapatellar tendon is obliterated.

Grade III. This is not done manually but is performed by placing a 4 in × 4 in × 6 in wooden block under the tibia with the patient in the supine position and the knee extended. This passively demonstrates the integrity of the ACL because the femur descends below the tibia from the weight of the upper leg if there is incompetence of the ACL. During the second portion of the test, the block is placed under the lower end of the femur and the tibial tuberosity ascends. The infrapatellar fossa is observed from the side (Fig. 4–12).

Grade IV. With the patient seated, the quadriceps is actively and forcefully contracted. In the presence of a torn ACL, the tibia translates forward (subluxation) (Fig 4–13).

Rotatory instability can also be tested as indicated in Figure 4–14. This supplements the Lachman test.

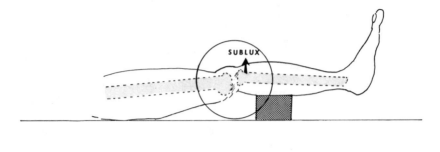

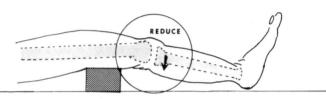

Figure 4–12. Wooden block test for ACL inadequacy. With the patient lying supine, a 4 in × 4 in × 6 in block is placed under the tibia. If there is ACL inadequacy, the femur descends and the infrapatellar space is obliterated, indicating anterior subluxation of the tibia (a tear of the ACL). Placing the block under the femur reduces the subluxation and places the support upon the posterior cruciate ligament.

Mechanism of ACL Injury

Injury to the ACL occurs commonly from a forceful valgus external rotational injury (Figs. 4–15 and 4–16). An injury to the ACL that occurs by this mechanism is often associated with damage to other medial supporting structures such as the medial collateral ligaments. An isolated injury to the ACL can result from forceful internal rotation of the femur with or without significant extension. In this maneuver, the ligament impinges at the anterior aspect of the intercondylar notch.[15]

Downhill skiing or similiar athletic activities that require a flexed knee position with a subsequent passive posterior drawer motion and a forceful quadriceps contraction can result in damage to the ACL.

Diagnosis of ACL Injury

Injury to the ligament is frequently noticed by the injured individual who hears an audible "snap" sound. In most patients this is followed by an acute effusion; severe, profound disability; and painful limited range of motion of the knee. Examination, even at a very early stage, becomes difficult and uninformative because of the effusion, which limits the value of

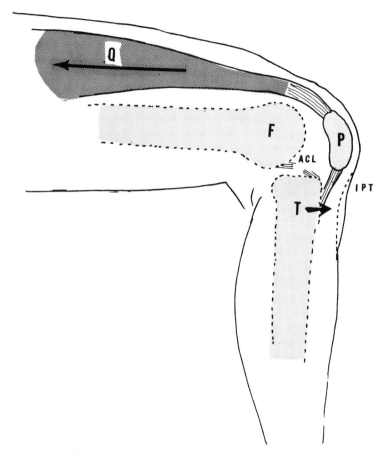

Figure 4–13. Quadriceps test of a grade III ACL inadequacy. In the seated position with the knee at a 45° angle, forceful contraction of the quadriceps will anteriorly sublux the tibia if the ACL is torn. This subluxation can be easily seen.

a drawer test and even of a Lachman test, although the latter is more accurate. Examination under anesthesia and after aspiration of the hemarthrosis is valuable.

The presence of effusion and/or hemarthrosis may escape the examiner if the effusion is relatively minor. Confirmation of the presence of effusion is obtained by using the ballottement test (Fig. 4–17). Downward pressure on the suprapatellar space forces the fluid under the patella, giving a positive ballottement test, while downward pressure on the patella may merely dispel the fluid and give a false negative test.

Joint effusion causes quadriceps paresis from a neurological reflex basis[16] and should, for this reason, be removed or diminished early.

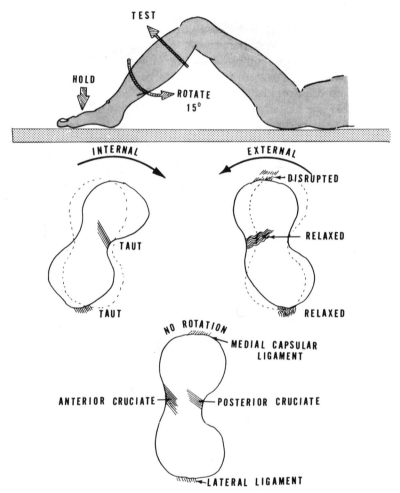

Figure 4–14. Rotatory instability test. A recumbent patient is examined with knee and hip flexed to 90°. Examiner sits on plantigrade foot (hold). Tibia is examined with 15° internal, no rotation, then 15° external rotation. The examiner pulls tibia forward upon the femur (test). With tibia *externally* rotated, the anterior cruciate ligament is relaxed as are the lateral ligaments. Excessive anterior displacement indicates medial capsular disruption (a positive test). With tibia *internally* rotated forward, movement of tibia upon femur is limited by posterolateral capsule, posterior cruciate ligament, fibular collateral ligament, and popliteus tendon and tensor fascia lata (not shown). With tibia *externally* rotated, the test is to determine adequacy of (1) medial capsular ligament, (2) anterior portion of medial collateral ligament, and (3) ultimately, the anterior cruciate ligament (if 1 and 2 are torn).

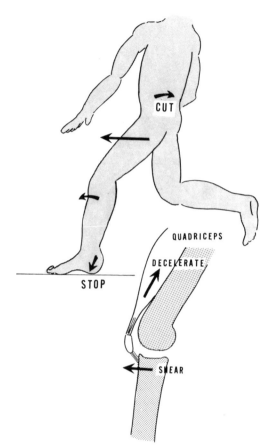

Figure 4–15. "Stop and cut" mechanism of athletic injury. Coming to an abrupt stop, with or without simultaneous rotation (cut) places shear stress on the knee. The quadriceps abruptly decelerates the knee flexion, placing added shear stress on the knee. Added "cut" adds rotatory stress upon the knee. Quadriceps deceleration causes anterior cruciate ligament shear. Deceleration is the "culprit."

Treatment of ACL Disruption

The "natural history" of knees suffering a disruption of the ACL remains unclear. This affects statistical evaluation of treatment procedures. In most clinical studies the prognosis of ACL tears treated nonsurgically is subjectively favorable. Most injured patients return to athletic activities but to what extent, intensity, and duration is not clear. The "quality of life" remains undefined.

Prognosis also varies as regards the degree of ligamentous tear. A partially torn ACL has a more favorable prognosis than does a completely torn one,[17] but it is also difficult to document the degree of injury. Current prospective arthroscopic examination studies may provide better prognostic determinations.

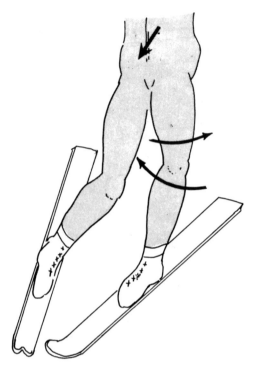

Figure 4–16. Mechanism of rotatory knee injury. As an example, a skier on downward glide (thick arrow) twists body to the left. The left ski does not rotate. The leg at the knee externally rotates the femur upon the tibia.

Because of associated injuries in other ligaments and/or the meniscus that usually accompany this ligamentous injury, there is a high rate of early degenerative arthritic changes. Stability usually remains sufficiently adequate to permit return to preinjury activities, but many patients admit to a decrease in athletic activities.

GENERAL TREATMENT OF LIGAMENTOUS INJURIES

Mild Sprain

Pain can be elicited by applying stress to the ligaments. There is usually tenderness over the collateral ligaments and some local swelling is noted, but there is no effusion. The joint is stable. Active movements of the knee may be painful and limited.

Treatment is essentially the relief of discomfort through the application of ice packs for 20 minutes several times a day. Compression dressings limit knee motion and decrease further effusion. Oral nonsteroidal anti-inflammatory medication may be palliative. Injection of an anesthetic agent

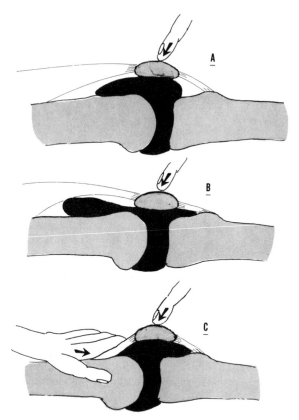

Figure 4–17. Ballottement test for effusion. (*A*) Fluid may not be visible and downward pressure upon the patella causes no ballottement. (*B*) The fluid disperses upward under the suprapatellar tendon and downward under the infrapatellar tendon. With small amounts of fluid, this procedure does not confirm the presence of significant fluid (a negative ballottement test), nor does it facilitate aspiration. (*C*) Downward pressure upon the suprapatellar tendon displaces the fluid from the suprapatellar bursa and causes medial lateral bulging of the capsule. This permits a positive ballottement of the patella that confirms the presence of fluid (blood) and facilitates aspiration.

with or without steroids is usually not needed. Resumption of activities may be left to the judgment of the patient.

Moderate Sprain

Local swelling and some effusion, which can be elicited by ballottement (Fig. 4–17), are noted. Pain is elicited by actively stressing the joint, and the

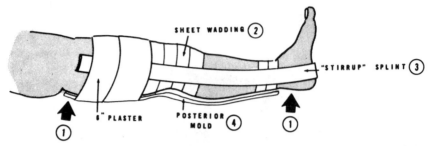

Figure 4–18. Method of pressure dressing and casting. The leg is held behind the thigh and the heel (*1*) to permit the tibia to hang, thus relaxing the anterior cruciate ligament. The first wrap is a sheet wadding (or gauze) (*2*) for uniform compression. A stirrup splint made of plaster strips (*3*) is used to prevent lateral motion. A posterior mold splint (*4*) with the foot dorsiflexed is then applied, and a final wraparound of gauze or 6 inches of a thin layer of plaster is used.

range of motion is limited. Locking occurs if there is meniscal involvement. A "soggy" limitation may reveal ACL involvement on Lachman manuever, but the presence of effusion makes this determination unreliable.

Treatment consists of bed rest, an external orthosis (canvas brace), and the use of crutches during ambulation. Elevation of the limb and application of ice packs are necessary. Pressure dressing is demonstrated in Figure 4–18.

Aspiration is valuable in determining whether there is effusion or hemarthrosis. Aspiration decreases pain and makes further examination possible. There are both mechanical and histological reasons[18] for aspirating the blood in the joint. In joint blood, there are iron-laden synovial and subsynovial macrophages that produce degenerative enzymes that can damage joint cartilage. These changes as well as the elongation of the joint ligaments and capsules of the knee joint caused by the presence of the fluid mandate that the hemorrhage be removed early and repeatedly (if there is recurrence).

The duration of immobilization is conjectural; 3 weeks is usually recommended. *During immobilization, frequent isometric quadriceps contraction exercises should be prescribed.* This enhances dispersal of the effusion and minimizes subsequent quadriceps atrophy. Electrical stimulation of the quadriceps may enhance recovery.

Severe Sprain

In severe sprain some ligaments are torn. These may be the cruciates, either of the collaterals, or all three. Disability is severe and immediate. Effusion may actually be hemarthrosis, which can be determined by aspiration *under sterile conditions.* The details of the diagnosis and treatment of these ligaments have been discussed.

In a severe ligamentous injury implying significant tibiofemoral subluxation, vascular and/or neurological injury may occur and should be suspected and verified. The posterior popliteal artery is attached superiorly to the femur by a tendinous hiatus within the adductor magnus muscle, which permits no mobility. The artery then descends beneath the tendinous arch of the soleus, where it is attached firmly to the tibia. Any shear motion of the tibia on the femur can injure the artery (Fig. 4–19). The common peroneal nerve can also be injured in a knee subluxation injury.

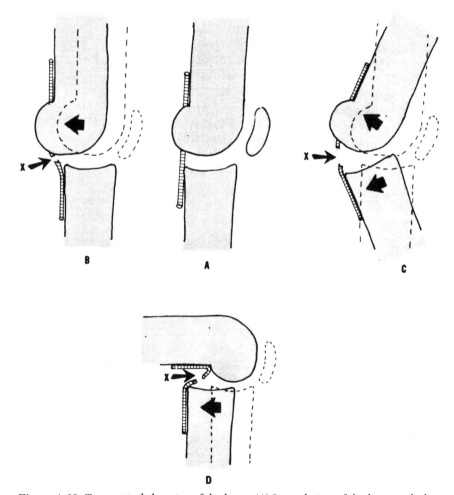

Figure 4–19. Traumatic dislocation of the knee. (A) Lateral view of the knee with the popliteal artery adherent to the lower femur and the upper tibia. (B) Direct injury to the femur, causing posterior luxation (shear) with arterial tear, (X). (C) Hyperextension injury. (D) Common auto accident injury with flexed knee, causing the tibia to dislocate posteriorly. Here also there is a blood vessel injury.

Braces

Bracing an injured ACL has long been advocated to support the knee and to permit resumption of athletic activities. More recently, bracing has been advocated to prevent knee injuries in athletic activities that commonly cause direct knee trauma.

Effective braces for the patient who has sustained an ACL injury are available, but their use in resumption of strenuous athletic activites is limited. Biomedical studies indicate that most braces of current design limit rotatory mobility (hence guard against further instability in an ACL-injured knee) but fail to significantly decrease translation of the tibia on the femoral condyles. Essentially low-load activities are permitted, but high-load activities remain equivocal.

There also remains controversy as to the efficacy of currently available braces in preventing ligamentous injury.[19] Questions concerning the benefit of prophylactic braces are: How do braces perform under impact situations? Do they give the athlete a false sense of security, hence decreasing the effectiveness of other methods of prevention.

The American Academy of Orthopaedic Surgeons (AAOS) has questioned the terms "brace" and "guard" and has favored the former.[25] The term "brace" indicates an orthosis in which there is a metal or plastic bar across the knee which limits unwanted movement from external forces. The usual brace protects the medial knee ligamentous structures from lateral forces. The brace must extend from above the knee joint at the lower thigh and to the upper calf area. A hinge that permits flexion must be included.

Several physiological factors justify braces that stabilize the knee against valgus from lateral forces acting on the knee joint. The medial collateral ligament, especially its long fibers,[20] acts as a tether to oppose excessive valgus opening of the inner aspect of the knee. The MCL is at its greatest elongation when the knee is completely extended, the greatest tension being at the anterior long fibers.[21]

There are other tissues that stabilize the knee against excessive valgus: the sartorius, gracilis, semitendinosus, and vastus medialis muscles. It has been shown that the knee becomes more stable when there is contraction of the vastus medialis and sartorius muscles preceding a lateral force.[22] The semimembranosus muscle tendon complex (Fig. 4–20) is probably the most efficient corollary supporting structure by virtue of its triple insertion design that spans the entire medial tibiofemoral joint space. The vastus medialis portion of the quadriceps muscle also plays a part in medial knee support.

Proprioceptive reflexes allegedly act to minimize impact on ligaments by reflex contraction of the protective muscles. This has been refuted[23] since apparently an adequate reflex does not exist in the MCL, and even if it would respond, the response is too slow to prevent injury.[24]

Normal valgus of the knee, predicted by the degree of the Q angle, preloads the MCL and "stiffens" the knee. In a brace that decreases this angle, the effect is diminished or lost.

The brace is structured to prevent severe valgus stretching or tearing of the medial collateral ligaments (Fig. 4–21). The lateral bar of the brace must be sufficiently far away from the joint so as to prevent valgus and not touch the joint when there is excessive lateral force. The brace also must not slip

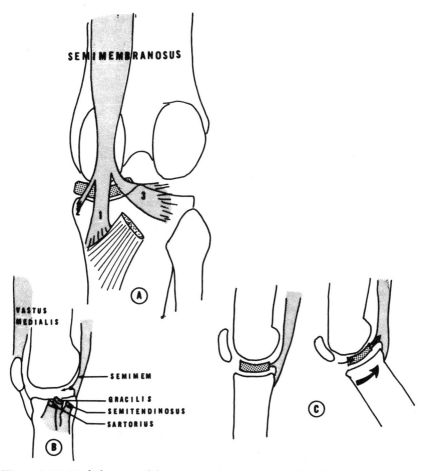

Figure 4–20. Medial aspect of the posterior knee structure. (A) The semimembranosus muscle has four tendinous inserts. The major insert (1) extends to attach on the posterior aspect of the tibia and sends fibers into the popliteus. In its path there is an exterior branch that attaches to the posterior aspect of the medial meniscus (2 and 3). These tendons complete the posterior popliteal fossa and tense the capsule. (B) The medial aspect of the knee with the insertion sites of the medial flexors. (C) The semimembranosus flexes the knee and simultaneously pulls the meniscus backward and rotates it with the tibia.

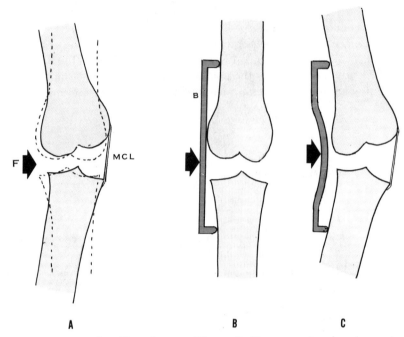

Figure 4–21. Principles of knee bracing. The vertical bar prevents valgus (*arrow* in A) causing strain upon the medial collateral ligament (MCL). The bar (*B*) absorbs the impact. If the metal of the brace is too flexible, it bends (*C*) and allows valgus.

downward, changing the balance of forces and altering the site of the knee joint. Lateral force may also cause rotation if the force is applied when the knee is slightly bent, causing stress to be imposed on the cruciates rather than on the collateral ligaments.

Numerous studies have attempted to determine the efficacy of preventative bracing. Teitz[26] found no advantage. The AAOS also found no advantage; the AAOS actually found that athletes using a knee brace had more knee, foot, and ankle injuries.[25] Other studies found benefit from prophylactic braces.

These studies have been refuted by claiming that the brace originally was to prevent only collateral ligament injury and that the value of the brace depends on the position and thus the activities of the athlete wearing the brace. The consensus is that more research and better construction of the brace is needed.

Miscra, Daniel, and Stone[27] studied the efficacy and complaints of the wearers of Don Joy 4 Point, RKS, Lenox Hill, and CTi. They found that when the braces are worn, there is no "giving away of the knee" and limited pivotal shift. Anterior displacement was measured and found to be diminished. Many of those tested complained of limited activities during squatting and full deep knee bends, some downward slipping of the brace, and a feeling of "bulkiness" in athletic equipment.

Following surgery to repair ACL, investigators have noted a significant quadriceps insufficiency[27] that adds to knee instability. Atrophy initially occurs within the first 7 to 14 days postoperatively, which is the period of immobilization following surgery. After one year this insufficiency has not usually been regained. A neurological reason has been propounded, and it also indicates the need for an aggressive postoperative quadriceps physical therapy program.

There is concomitant atrophy and weakness of the quadriceps and hamstring muscles following ACL disruption, and this forms the basis for initiating an immediate exercise program. In the case of surgical intervention for repair of the ACL, 2 weeks of postoperative casting is usual, and within those weeks atrophy occurs. The loss of quadriceps strength is greater than that of the hamstring muscle groups, but both occur and persist after injury.

It is a well-accepted fact that immediately after a knee injury, especially if there is effusion, a reflex inhibition of contraction of the quadriceps occurs. This has been postulated as a reflex neurological inhibition mediated through the spindle system. Regardless of the neurological basis, the injured patient usually cannot contract the quadriceps, thus electrical stimulation during isometric contraction should be initiated. Electrical stimulation enhances the contraction[28] and possibly initiates the concept of contraction long before the patient can initiate voluntary contraction. It has also been noted that the strength deficits were greater in the high-speed than in the low-speed kinetic testings, allegedly due to the atrophy being more common in the type II muscle fibers.[29]

The deficiency of the ACL-injured knee is anterolateral subluxation producing a painful "giving way" of the knee during physical activities. Only strengthening of the quadriceps and the hamstring muscle can diminish this action in daily activities. The hamstrings especially perform this activity because they are agonists of the ACL. Because the loss is in the high-speed rather than in the low-speed muscle fibers, this should be considered in prescribing resistance exercises.

Observation of the loss of bulk should be noted, especially in the vastus medialis oblique muscle group, as there is a greater tendency for atrophy to be evident in that group of muscles. Weakness is also noted in the last 15° to 30° of extension.

Tightness may result and remain in the hamstring muscle group (Figs. 4–22 and 4–23) and in the quadriceps, which should be released by gradual, progressive stretching exercises.[30]

Arthroscopic studies have noted a significant degree of cartilaginous changes, though they are initially asymptomatic. Further follow-up studies are needed to see if, in later years, these changes become symptomatic. Degenerative arthritis of the knee is discussed further in Chapter 6.

"PROTECTIVE" HAMSTRING STRETCH

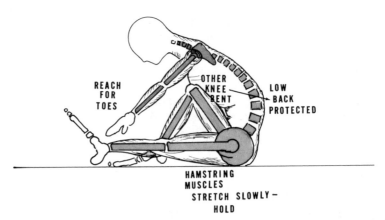

Figure 4–22. Protective hamstring muscle stretch. The lower back is protected when this gentle, progressive stretch is performed. With one leg flexed and placed to the chest, there is minimal stretch of the low back, while the other extended leg undergoes a gradual stretch of the hamstring. With very limited extension of both hamstrings, resistance is compensated by an excessive low-back stretch, which may aggravate low-back symptoms.

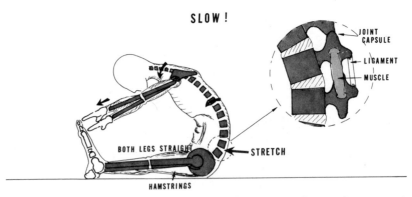

Figure 4–23. Bilateral hamstring muscle stretch exercise. This gentle, progressive bilateral hamstring stretch must be done slowly, gently, and gradually, with no "bounce." Both hamstrings, which consist of six muscles, may overwhelm the lower back (see insert) if the exercise is done rapidly and violently; hence, the admonition of doing the exercise *slowly.*

REFERENCES

1. Cailliet, R: Soft Tissue Pain and Disability, ed 2. FA Davis, Philadelphia, 1988.
2. Thomas, CL (ed): Taber's Cyclopedic Medical Dictionary, ed 15. FA Davis, Philadelphia, 1985.
3. Brantigan, OC and Voshell, AF: Mechanics of ligaments and menisci of the knee joint. J Bone Joint Surg 23:43, 1941.
4. Torg, JS, Conrad, W, and Kalen, V: Clinical diagnosis of anterior cruciate ligament instability in the athlete. Am J Sports Med 4:84, 1976.
5. Grood, ES, et al: Ligamentous and capsular restraints preventing straight medial and lateral laxity in intact human cadaver knees. J Bone Joint Surg 63A:1257, 1981.
6. Kennedy, JC and Fowler, PJ: Medial and anterior instability of the knee: An anatomical and clinical study using stress machines. J Bone Joint Surg 53A:1257, 1971.
7. Indelicato, PA: Nonoperative management of complete tears of the medial collateral ligament. Pain Management 263, vol XVIII September/October 1990.
8. Kannus, P: Long-term results of conservatively treated medial collateral ligament injuries of the knee joint. Clin Orthop 226:103, 1988.
9. Taylor, AR, Arden, GP, and Rainey, HA: Traumatic dislocation of the knee. J Bone Joint Surg 54B:96, 1972.
10. Meyers, MH and Harvey, JP: Traumatic dislocation of the knee joint: A study of eighteen cases. J Bone Joint Surg 53A:16, 1971.
11. Harrison, R and Hidenach, JC: Dislocation of the upper end of the fibula. J Bone Joint Surg 41B, 1959.
12. Snook, GA: A short history of the anterior cruciate ligament and the treatment of tears. Clin Orthop 172:11, 1983.
13. Gurtier, RA, Stine, R, and Torg, JS: Lachman test revisited. Contemporary Orthop 20(2):145, 1990.
14. Rebman, LW: Lachman's test: An alternative method. J Orthop Sports Phys Therap 9(11):381, 1988.
15. Bessette, GC and Hunter, RE: The anterior cruciate ligament: Review article. Orthopedics 13(5):551, 1990.
16. Arnoczky, SP, et al: Microvasculature of the cruciate ligaments and its response to injury: An experimental study in dogs. J Bone Joint Surg 61A:1221, 1979.
17. Odensten, M, Lysholm, J, and Gillquist, J: The course of partial injuries of the knee joint. Am J Sports Med 13(3):183, 1985.
18. Parsons, JR, Zingler, BM, and McKeon, JJ: Mechanical and histological studies of acute joint hemorrhage. Orthopedics 10(7):1019, 1987.
19. Russell, JA: The prophylactic knee guard controversy. Surg Rounds Orthop 27, July, 1990.
20. Warren, JF, Marshall, JI, and Girgis, F: The prime static stabilizer of the medial side of the knee. J Bone Joint Surg 56A(4):665, 1974.
21. Kennedy, JC, Hawkins, RJ, and Willis, RB: Strain gauge analysis of knee ligaments. Clin Orthop 129:225, 1977.
22. Pope, MH, et al: The role of the musculature in injuries to the medial collateral ligament. J Bone Joint Surg 61A(3):398, 1979.
23. Petersen, I and Stener, B: Experimental evaluation of the hypothesis of ligamentomuscular protective reflexes. III: A study in man using the medial collateral ligament of the knee joint. Acta Physiolo Scand (Suppl 166)48:51, 1959.
24. France, EP, et al: The biomechanics of lateral knee bracing. II: Impact response of the braced knee. Am J Sports Med 15(5):430, 1987.
25. American Academy of Orthopaedic Surgeons: Knee braces: seminar report. Park Ridge, Il. American Academy of Orthopaedic Surgeons, 1985.
26. Teitz, CC, Hermanson BK, et al: Evaluation of the use of braces to prevent injury to the knee in collegiate football players. J Bone Joint Surg 69A(1):2–9, 1987.

27. Miscra, DK, Daniel, DM, and Stone, ML: The use of functional knee braces in control of pathological anterior knee laxity. Clin Orthop Related Res 241:213, 1989.
28. LoPresti, C, et al: Quadriceps insufficiency following repair of the anterior cruciate ligament. J Orthop Sports Phys Therap 9(7):245, 1988.
29. Williams, RA, Morrissey, MC, and Brewster, CE: The effect of electrical stimulation on quadriceps strength and thigh circumference in meniscectomy patients. J Orthop Sports Phys Therap 8(3):143, 1986.
30. Kannus, P, Latvala, K, and Jarvinen, M: Thigh muscle strengths in the anterior cruciate ligament deficient knee: Isokinetic and isometric long term results. J Orthop Sports Phys Therap 9(6):223, 1987.
31. Antich, TJ, et al: Physical therapy treatment of knee extensor mechanism disorders: Comparison of four treatment modalities. J Orthop Sports Phys Therap 8(5):255, 1986.

CHAPTER 5

Patellofemoral Pain
and Impairment

Pathologies of the patellofemoral joint are considered to be a major cause of anterior knee pain. The patellofemoral joint was originally unrecognized in orthopedic literature. However, damage to this joint now constitutes a major disease entity in the complaint of anterior knee pain and impairment. Numerous diagnostic labels have emerged: the diagnosis "chondromalacia patellae" predominantly implicates the cartilage of the inner surface of the patella as the major source of anterior knee pain. In 1985 Radin[1] focused on the need for a precise diagnosis of anterior knee pain in his provocative article, "Anterior Knee Pain. The Need for a Specific Diagnosis: Stop Calling It Chondromalacia!" He further commented on the numerous surgical procedures advocated for the relief of knee pain with the statement, "Few orthopedic surgeons are happy with their treatment of patients with 'chondromalacia' of the patella."[2]

The theories and claims regarding the patella—its function, structure, pathology, and management—are numerous. Patients with anterior knee pain present a challenge, and appropriate, effective treatment remains an enigma, while revealing the perplexing problems presented by the patellofemoral joint and its components. Haxton[3] aptly presented the problem when he stated, "It seems likely that more has been written about the patella, relative to its size, than about any other bone in the human body."

FUNCTIONAL ROLE OF THE PATELLA

The role of the patella has been analyzed biomechanically (Fig. 5–1) in a parallelogram analysis and clinically in an evaluation of knee function in its absence. Bruce[4] claimed that the patella was unnecessary on the basis of

143

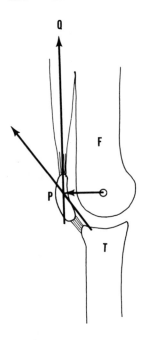

Figure 5–1. Parallelogram analysis of knee joint. Parallelogram of force from quadriceps (Q) action through the patella (P), a sesamoid bone that angles force from the femoral (F) alignment to attach to and extend the tibia (T).

follow-up of patellectomy patients. Scott[5] refuted this statement by revealing that only 5 percent of patients following a patellectomy functioned "normally." There is also a literature report[6] that quadriceps strength decreased 49 percent, knee flexion decreased, quadriceps atrophied significantly, and the total range of motion decreased by 18°.

The patella, a sesamoid bone contained "within" the quadriceps tendon, has asymmetrical facets on its inferior surface that are separated by a central ridge (Fig. 5–2). This surface is covered with cartilage and articulates in an incongruous manner with the femoral condyles, which are also coated with cartilage. When the tibiofemoral joint moves, the patella moves "with" the tibia about a vertical axis on the articular condyles of the femur.

When the patella moves on the femoral condyles, the contact sites (Fig. 5–3) vary depending on the precise degree of flexion-extension. The weight-bearing sites are depicted in this figure at varying degrees of flexion-extension. This has been discussed in Chapter 2. It may be noted that there is *no* weight bearing on the odd facet, which is located on the extreme medial aspect of the patella.

The cartilage of the patella has received a great deal of attention and has been considered to have the greatest degree of pathological significance. Because the patellar cartilage has also been singled out as *the* cause and site of anterior knee pain, its innervation should be considered.

The knee joint is supplied by a large number of articular twigs from muscular nerve branches emanating from the femoral, obturator, tibial, and

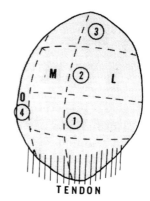

Figure 5–2. Facets of patella. The cartilaginous surface of the patella has a broader lateral (L) facet than a medial (M) one. Each half (M-L) is divided into three facets with the inferior facet attaching the infrapatellar tendon. The bottom drawing depicts the medial (M), lateral (L), and odd (O) facets from a superior view.

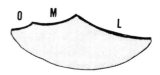

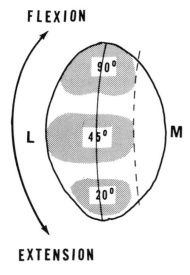

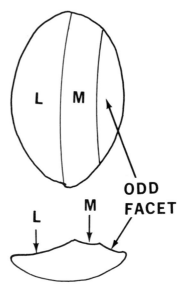

Figure 5–3. Contact site of the patella during flexion. (*Left*) Sites and area of contact of the patella to the femoral condyles during flexion of 20°, 45°, and 90°. The lateral (L) facets make contact through entire flexion-extension with no contact with the medial (M) or odd facets during physiological tracting.

common peroneal nerves. The articular branches of the femoral nerve to the knee joint arise from the saphenous nerve and the nerve going to the three vasti muscles. A branch from the nerve to the vastus intermedius goes to the suprapatellar aspect of the joint. A branch from the obturator nerve follows the femoral and popliteal arteries and goes to the posteromedial part of the capsule. The tibial nerve sends branches that accompany the genicular arteries, and a branch of the common peroneal nerve innervates the anterolateral part of the capsule. A recurrent branch of the peroneal nerve is distributed to the periosteum of the surface of the tibia and the tibiofibular joint. The horns of the menisci are well innervated, but the bodies of the menisci are not. The ligaments are also well innervated.[7]

Throughout the body all cartilage is avascular, alymphatic, and aneural. Since cartilage is devoid of innervation, any injury to it will not be appreciated until there is a synovial reaction. Since the synovium is innervated it transmits nociception. Pain can also be experienced when the cartilage has undergone sufficient degeneration to expose the underlying bone, which is also innervated and transmits pain. Structural damage to cartilage can therefore occur even though the patient is totally oblivious of the injury.

The mechanics of joints has been well documented,[8] and more recently the relationship of biomechanical and chemical degradation of cartilage to mechanical trauma has been better understood.[9] In his excellent article, Mankin[10] has discussed the reaction of articular cartilage to injury and osteoarthritis. The mechanism and diagnosis of degenerative osteoarthritis can be postulated based on these conclusions.

Since cartilage is avascular and alymphatic, nutrition destined for the cartilage must first diffuse out of the synovial vascular plexus, traverse the synovial membrane to enter the synovial fluid, and then pass through the dense hyaline matrix of the cartilage. Whereas before bone maturation cartilage can receive nutrition by diffusion through the basal layers from underlying bone, the vessels become occluded when the bone epiphysis ossifies. The final destiny of the nutrient is the chondrocyte.

The chondrocytes are sparse and were originally considered to be effete once the cartilage reached maturity. By virtue of newer electron microscopy studies, chondrocytes have been shown to be metabolically active.[11]

The matrix, which supplies the mechanical hydrodynamic support of the cartilage, is hyperhydrated, having 80 percent water bound to the proteoglycans of the tissue. Throughout the matrix are collagen fibrils (Fig. 5–4) that give mechanical support. The macromolecules of the matrix are bonded to the collagen fibrils, giving them resiliency and resistance to deformation. The cartilage under alternating pressure and relaxation imbibes the nutrient synovial material.

The chondrocytes are currently considered to be responsible for matrix turnover and renewal. Lysosomal enzymes, which are believed to be produced within the matrix, initiate turnover and renewal of matrix proteoglycans synthesized by the chondrocytes.

Structural and chemical responses to laceration injuries of the cartilage have been microscopically studied. Immediately after a laceration injury, there is a burst of mitotic activity within the cartilage that is immediately adjacent to the tear. This indicates an attempt at resynthesis, but this activity is short-lived, lasting approximately 1 week. There appears to be no relevant evidence of repair in further studies of these lacerated tissues.

Superficial lacerations neither heal nor progress. However, deep lacerations react differently. A condition termed "basal" degeneration has been described from arthrotomies and arthroscopies. This basal degeneration occurs in the "deep" layers of the cartilage, although the superficial surface is spared. This basal condition allegedly begins with fasciculation of a small segment of collagen fibers, with the immediate adjacent fibers remaining intact. The distal portion of the affected fibers deteriorates, and a "blister" forms, which ultimately ruptures and causes a fissure on the surface to the subchondral bone.

The site of basal degeneration with a resultant blister is claimed to occur at the ridge between the odd facet and the medial facet (see Fig. 5–2), which

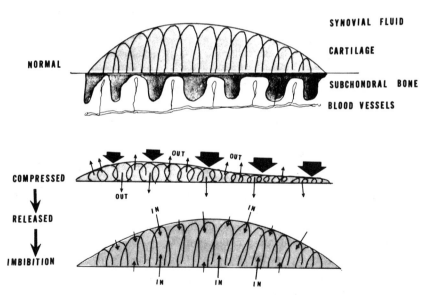

Figure 5–4. Normal cartilage metabolism. (*Top*) Normal cartilage with collagen fibrils within matrix upon subchondral bone (schematic). Nutrition comes from influx of synovial fluid and dialysate of bone blood vessels. (*Middle*) Pressure exudes hyaluronidase, mucin, chondroitin sulphate, and so forth from cartilage into synovial cavity and into bone blood vessels. (*Bottom*) Imbibition of nutrient fluids from release of compression of cartilage.

is the site of maximum pressure when the knee is flexed to 90° (see Fig. 5–3). This painful flexed knee condition is frequently noted in young people when weight is lifted with the knee flexed or when ascending stairs. This anterior knee pain occurs on arising after prolonged sitting with the knee at 90°. Full extension of the knee may relieve the pain.

A deep laceration into the basal layers, causing direct contact with the underlying bone end plate, may result in an evasion of vascular activity. This deep laceration immediately becomes filled with blood and elicits cellular enzymatic elements. Fibroblasts in this blood infiltrate, gradually producing a fibrocartilaginous mass. The cartilage distal from the bone end plate does not undergo repair nor is it covered by the more superficial layers. Years after the injury, the superficial laceration remains unchanged.

Because some injuries to the knee can simultaneously initiate a hemarthrosis and cartilaginous damage, the effect of blood in the synovial fluid and its effect on cartilage healing have been studied. A single episode of hemarthrosis causes *no* variation in chondrocyte activity.

Within 2 hours of a direct blow to the patella, there is an increase in free arachidonic acid concentration within the cartilage. This implies that trauma to the cartilage releases algogenic substances which are polypeptides known as kinins which, per se, are capable of causing pain. Damage to the cartilage also liberates phospholipid A2 which breaks down into arachidonic acid which further breaks down to prostaglandin PGE2 and PGF3. Arachidonic acid is a normal component of cellular phospholipids which, after trauma, are liberated by kinins. The prostaglandins that ultimately form digest the cartilage initiating a softening and fibrillation (Fig. 5–5). A significant quantity of released kinins produce additional enzymic synovitis resulting in a cascade effect.[12]

In this case, the synovium of the knee joint undergoes inflammatory invasion, predominantly of monocytes and lymphocytes. The synovium thickens from a one- or two-layer tissue to a tissue of five or more layers, and the subsynovial layer of fat becomes invaded with blood vessels. All these changes are an inflammatory reaction to the emergence of the proteoglycans that have resulted from trauma. These changes do *not* fit the definition of "inflammation" because normal cartilage has no blood supply; however, there is, without question, a biochemical inflammatory reaction. The enzymes are "cathepsins," which lyse proteins.[13] Injection of homogenized damaged cartilage into normal joints reproduced these changes, which are similar to osteoarthritic synovitis and degeneration.[14]

The term "chondromalacia" was initially credited to Aleman in 1917 by Karlson[15] but first appeared in the English medical literature in 1933.[16] From that time on, all anterior knee pain involving the patella was termed "chondromalacia" without necessarily being specific about whether it was primary or secondary to other knee pathology. Chondromalacia has been repeatedly discovered in totally asymptomatic adult knees.[17]

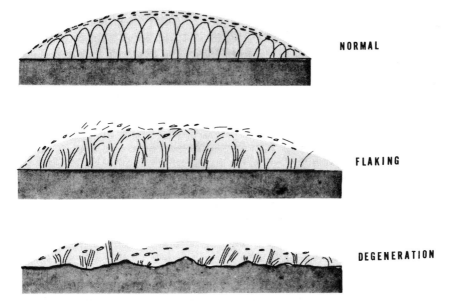

NORMAL

FLAKING

DEGENERATION

Figure 5–5. Stages of degenerative arthritis.

Current concepts postulate that chondromalacia may be latent from repeated multiple microtraumata and become symptomatic after a greater trauma. The repeated microtraumata are possibly repetitive, or there is prolonged loading force on the cartilage, which compresses the tissue and causes decreased elasticity with diminution of nutrition of the cartilage. Abnormal anatomic relationships between the patella and the femoral condyles predispose the knee to chondromalacia and ultimate osteoarthritic changes.

The stages of chondromalacia[18] are established as being (1) swelling and softening of the cartilage, possibly from superficial laceration incurred from trauma that progresses or occurs simultaneously with (2) fissuring of the softened portion of the cartilage and (3) surface deformation termed fasciculation (see Fig. 5–5). These three stages are stages of chondromalacia. A later stage (4), termed "osteoarthritis," can be considered to occur when the (deep) fissuring reaches the subchondral bone with a vascular response. The first three stages may be asymptomatic or transiently symptomatic, which influences diagnosis and the resultant treatment.

It becomes apparent that precise diagnosis of the true basis of patellofemoral pain is difficult. Asymptomatic knees may already have beginning stages of chondromalacia that will become symptomatic when there is severe or repeated trauma, stage 3 is reached, or frank degenerative changes have occurred. An acute injury may present transient pain. A patellofemoral injury rarely evokes effusion. Spontaneous recovery may result before a specific diagnosis is made. Careful, meaningful examination is important in eliciting "potential" pathology in the early changes when there is suspicion of impending pathology.

The knee of the patient may "give out," may "click," or may momentarily "lock." Crepitation may be reported or noted on examination. Any "objective" change in patellar position, alignment, or tracking must be ascertained and addressed. These objective signs are:

1. Increase in quadriceps Q angle (see Fig. 2–13)
2. Laxity of the quadriceps tendon, as elicited by the patellar tilt test (Fig. 2–16), the seated tubercle-sulcus angle (Fig. 2–15), the patellar glide test (Fig. 2–17), or the lateral patellar pull test (Fig. 2–18)
3. A shallow patellar fossa established on x-ray
4. Abnormal inferior patellar contours
5. Patella alba
6. Excessive tibial torsion
7. Marked internal femoral torsion
8. Severe foot pronation
9. Secondary to internal femoral derangement such as anterior cruciate ligament tear and laxity, meniscal damage, and postoperative meniscectomy
10. Quadriceps inadequacy from whatever cause
11. Severe genu varus, valgus, or recurvatum
12. Symptomatic crepitation, elicited by comparing to result of similar pressure on the asymptomatic knee

Crepitation can be elicited (Fig. 5–6) by applying gentle downward and upward pressure on the patella while the patient carefully, slowly, and gently contracts the quadriceps. The application of "slow and gentle" pressure is important since pain can be elicited in a normal patellofemoral joint if this test is done abruptly and forcefully. The unaffected knee should be tested before the affected one so as to orient the patient to what is intended, to alleviate any concern on the part of the patient, and to provide a comparison with the afflicted knee.

RADIOLOGICAL EVALUATION

The first radiological method for visualizing the patellofemoral joint was described in 1921[19] and became prevalent in diagnosing anatomical pathological changes in the joint. Modification of this technique evolved[20] as depicted in Figure 5–7. Plain axial x-rays, however, have caused many questionable diagnostic interpretations because of image distortion, lack of standardization, and failure to ascertain the degree of femoral rotation. Also,

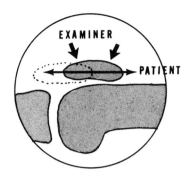

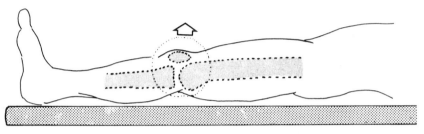

Figure 5–6. Examination for patellofemoral articulation. With leg extended and quadriceps relaxed, the examiner presses down upon the patella in a downward, then upward, direction. The patient then slowly contracts and relaxes the quadriceps; pain and crepitation may be elicited.

the need for visualizing the patellofemoral joint with the least amount of knee flexion (20° to 30°) has posed technical problems.[21]

   Computerized tomography (CT) scanning produces undistorted cross-sectional images at any degree of knee flexion. There are now criteria that standardize subluxation and patellar tilt.[22]

   Radionuclide imaging of the patellofemoral joint is being evaluated as a diagnostic technique for giving "objective" evidence of pathology and explaining the subjective complaint of anterior knee pain. Currently, imaging is in its infancy.[23] Arthrograms are not diagnostic, and arthroscopy is valuable for determining the presence and degree of articular superficial pathology. However, neither technique is accurate for determining incongruity of the patellofemoral components.

TREATMENT

   When the clinical and physical examinations, history, and appropriate radiological and nucleotide studies confirm the source of pain to be

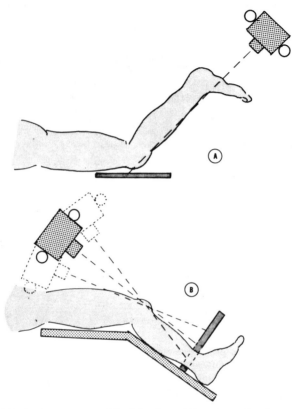

Figure 5–7. A technique suggested by Merchant (A) is claimed to be more accurate than the standard axial views taken at (B) 45° knee flexion, then 30° and 60°.

patellofemoral articular in etiology, appropriate treatment depends on the stage, duration, and severity of the injury.

The postulated sequence of early patellofemoral osteoarthritis is the basis for effective treatment protocol. In the acute stages, nonsteroidal medications, which are essentially prostaglandin synthesis inhibitors, delay or inhibit the production of prostaglandin B-2, which is the culprit in ultimate cartilage degeneration. Aspirin has been advocated by many, but others consider it of minimal value. The nonsteroidal drugs merit consideration if they are tolerated.

Patient education is mandatory if there is to be any benefit from a conservative treatment program. Once the patient understands how the patella can cause pain, be damaged, and gradually, even assuredly, become degenerated with osteoarthritis, adherence to the program will be enhanced. The patient will understand why ascending and descending stairs (Figs. 5–8 and 5–9), deep knee bends, kneeling, and prolonged sitting with

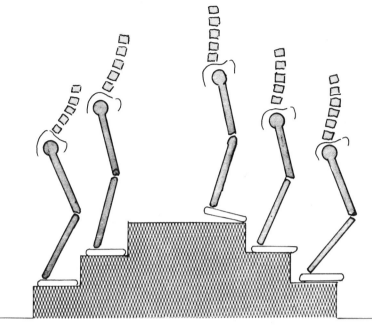

Figure 5–8. Knee in stair climbing and descending. As the person climbs the stairs, the knee flexes approximately 50° and the body leans forward; in descending, the body remains more erect above the hip joint with knee flexing to approximately 65°.

the knee in a flexed position must be avoided or minimized. When prolonged sitting is necessary, as in driving in a car, the patient should keep the knee extended as much as possible and preferably have it supported.

In the early acute phase, the knee should be rested. A cast or a velcro knee extensor brace should be avoided since both immobilize the knee and allow atrophy, which occurs rapidly. Local ice application (20 minutes q.i.d.) decreases pain, edema, and inflammation, and inhibits the formation of kinins, histamine, and nociceptor enzymes that accompany inflammation.

A knee support that permits full motion but prevents compression of the patella on the femoral condyles (Fig. 5–10) is indicated because it permits motion of the knee joint and quadriceps contraction, thus avoiding atrophy and minimizing joint contracture. The patella, guided by the brace, tracks in a physiological direction.

Quadriceps exercises, initially isotonic and then short-range extension contraction, should be instituted. If the pain is severe, isometric quadriceps contraction can be started. A slow maximum quadriceps isometric contraction should be held for 5 to 10 seconds and performed at least 50 times daily. When the pain decreases, the patient should progress to isometric contraction: straight leg raising with the weight on the lower leg increasing over

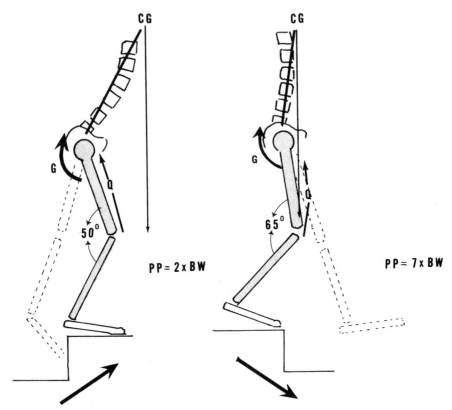

Figure 5–9. Patellar pressure in stair climbing and descending. (*Left*) Stair climbing. The knee flexes an average of 50° and the body leans forward, advancing the center of gravity (CG) and increasing the gluteal efficiency (G). The patellar pressure (PP) due to quadriceps contracture (Q) is two times the body weight (BW). (*Right*) Stair descending. The knee flexes an average of 65°, the body reclines backward of center of gravity, gluteal efficiency is decreased, and patellar pressure is seven times body weight. This is one of the factors resulting in patellar pain (chondromalacia).

time (Fig. 5–11). The beginning weight should be 10 pounds. The leg is raised to 45° and held for several seconds, with 10 repetitions. The weight should be gradually increased to 20 to 30 pounds. A lower back problem could be caused or aggravated if both legs are extended, so the opposite knee should always be flexed. The "weight" lifted can be a purse or shopping bag filled with increasing weight. Why quadriceps exercises help relieve patellofemoral pain remains unknown, but some reasons for the benefit may be (1) intermittent compression and relaxation of the patellar cartilage, (2) diffusion of the extra-articular nociceptive enzymes within the joint, (3) tightening of the parapatellar ligaments, or (4) production of endorphins.

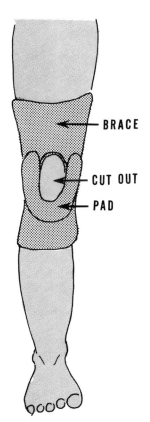

BRACE

CUT OUT

PAD

Figure 5–10. Knee brace for patellofemoral "tracking." The brace, which prevents patellofemoral malalignment, consists of an elastic-fitted webbing brace that is cut out over the patella with a pad around the medial, lateral, and inferior borders of the patella.

This custom-designed brace tracks the patella throughout flexion and extension of the knee.

Swimming exercises are of value because they offer active resistance and range of motion exercises without weight bearing. The hamstring muscles are usually ignored in knee rehabilitation, but, in the author's opinion, hamstring exercises (Fig. 5–12) help recovery. In 80 percent of patients with patellofemoral pain, a conscientiously followed, conservative program, as outlined, will result in recovery within 3 to 6 months.[24]

REFERRED PAIN

In every case of anterior knee pain, the possibility of referred pain from spinal radiculitis,[26] hip pathology, or intrinsic bone pathology must be ruled out. The complicating factors contributing to knee pain, such as severe valgus or varus, or severely pronated feet, must be recognized and addressed.

In 80 percent of patients with patellofemoral pain, a conservative

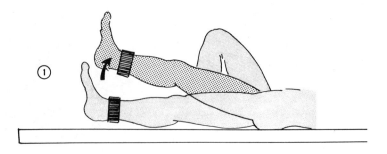

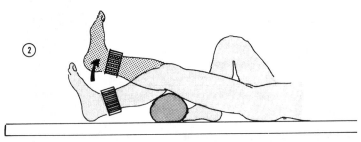

Figure 5–11. Quadriceps exercise for chondromalacia patella. (*1*) With leg extended and relaxed, the quadriceps is gently "tightened," the leg is lifted slowly to 45°, held there briefly, and then lowered. Once down, the quadriceps is relaxed. The opposite leg is flexed to "protect" the lower back. (*2*) The involved leg is flexed approximately 45° with a weight about the ankle (2 lb, then gradually to 10 to 15 lb). The leg is slowly extended—held—then slowly relaxed. Both (*1*) and (*2*) are done with 20 repetitions 3 to 5 times daily.

treatment program will result in recovery within 3 to 6 months.[24] These statistics are from patients without complicating factors of patellofemoral pathology, such as a significant synovial shelf, inflamed plica, osteochondritis dissecans, loose body, reflex sympathetic dystrophy, or meniscus tear. Referred pain, instead of intrinsic pathology, must be considered and ruled out. Stougard[25] presented the sobering facts of a poor correlation between gross chondromalacia and anterior knee pain and of studies that reveal negative arthroscopic studies in symptomatic patients.

Before considering surgical intervention, with its reported high incidence of failure, a definite preoperative diagnosis must be established. It is redundant to state that a careful history and a meaningful examination should be undertaken to document the presence and degree of patellar malalignment; limited patellar tilt, rigidity, or flexibility; and the presence of alba and excessive Q angle. Tenderness of the retinaculum must be ascertained by palpation of the peripatellar tissues to elicit the presence of a neuroma. Deep patellar tenderness consistent with a "jumper's knee" must be eliminated.

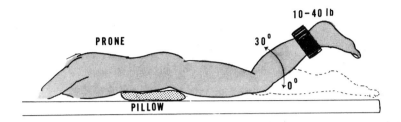

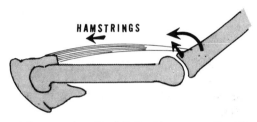

Figure 5–12. Hamstring exercise. (*Top*) Patient is prone with pillow under abdomen to decrease lordosis. Knee flexes slowly from full extension (0°) to 30°, beginning with 10 lb and increasing to 40 lb, repeating exercise 30 times each series. (*Bottom*) The hamstrings flex the knee and lightly shear the tibia posteriorly.

Confirmatory tests, such as computerized tomography, to determine patellofemoral tracking through the first 30° of flexion should be performed to substantiate clinical impression of inadequate tilting, lateral-medial shift, or segmental Q angle abnormal tracking. Routine x-rays are not reliable.

It is also mandatory that the conservative treatment regime be followed judiciously, carefully, and consistently for a reasonable time (3 months, but preferably 6 months). Evaluation and correction, whenever possible, of significant hip pathology, severe femoral and tibial torsion, severe foot pronation, and severe varus or valgus must precede surgical consideration, because they will interfere with and even negate surgical success.

SURGICAL INTERVENTION

There are numerous surgical procedures that have been advocated in treating the conditions of malalignment, patella alba, chondromalacia, and/or osteoarthritis of the patella. It is not the author's intent to discuss these techniques but merely to discuss the indications, contraindications, and presurgical and postsurgical care.

Gross malalignment is often treated by lateral release of the retinaculum[28] with mixed results. The conclusion of Kolowich and associates[27] is that a lateral release should be considered in patients with a negative patellar tilt, a medial or lateral glide of two quadrants or less, or a normal tubercle-sulcus angle. They considered a release to be questionable if there was a hypermobile patella that allowed subluxation, a positive passive patellar tilt, a medial lateral glide of greater than three quadrants, or an abnormal tubercle-sulcus angle. Merchant, in a discussion of this paper, stated that the "ideal" patient was one with a tight lateral tether (negative tilt), a normal Q angle, and a normal tubercle-sulcus angle. It is apparent from a review of the literature that only a tight patellar retinaculum with symptomatic patel-lofemoral arthralgia should be considered for a lateral release.

The tissue components of the anterior knee are depicted (Fig. 5–13) to show all the components that move the patella within the femoral condyles and that are normally at a slight lateral angle (Qa). The retinaculum places a mechanical restriction to medial shift and to excessive elevation of the lateral aspect of the patella (Fig. 5–14). With the quadriceps "pulling" the patella in at a slight angle (Qa) from a direct sagittal plane, the lateral and medial facets bear a proportionate amount of the compressive forces.

Significant retinaculum contracture (shortening) (Fig. 5–15) causes the retinaculum to thicken. The contained nerve (sensory) may form a painful neuroma. This shortening pulls the patella laterally, causing the lateral patellar facets to be excessively compressed, resulting in degeneration and gradual formation of degenerative arthritis.

Patients with an advanced malalignment appear to do less well after undergoing merely a lateral release which does not correct the gross subluxation or malalignment that has been the major cause of patellofemoral pain. When there has been a neuroma in the retinaculum causing pain, a lateral release apparently diminishes pain as it essentially denervates the neuroma (Fig. 5–16).

The patella that exhibits chronically malaligned tracking gradually undergoes adaptive re-formation (Wolff's law), which makes the "newly" shaped patella unable to adapt to the femoral condylar track. As stated, the lateral facet undergoes degenerative arthritic changes that lead to continuing painful activation. Lateral release is a good procedure if temporary benefit is expected and if the malalignment has been minor and brief in duration. Release or lengthening of the vastus lateralis muscle (see Fig. 5–13) enhances the resultant realignment of lateral release of the retinaculum.

Without a diligent, persistent, and intensive postoperative regime of exercise to regain quadriceps function, lateral retinacular release does not successfully relieve anterior knee pain and instability. The reasons why quadriceps strength and endurance are not regained remain unknown, but they are probably related to the failure to initiate a precise progressive regime prior to significant atrophy and to the absence of patient discipline and perseverance.

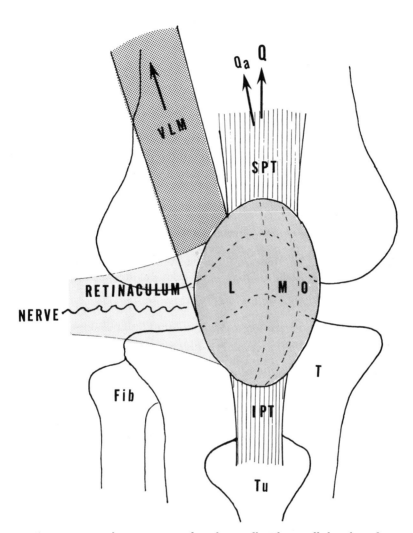

Figure 5–13. Anterior knee tissues guiding the patella. The patella has three facets on its inferior surface depicted as (L) lateral, (M) medial, and (O) odd. The quadriceps muscle (Q) attaches superiorly via the suprapatellar tendon (SPT) and attaches to the tibial tubercle (Tu) via the infrapatellar tendon (IPT). The extensor force of the quadriceps is in the direction of the quadriceps angle (Qa).

The vastus lateralis muscle (VLM) attaches obliquely to the patella and exerts lateral as well as superior force (*arrow*). The lateral retinaculum attaches to the lateral margin of the patella and exerts lateral stabilizing force. It contains a sensory nerve. (T) indicates tibia and (Fib) the fibula.

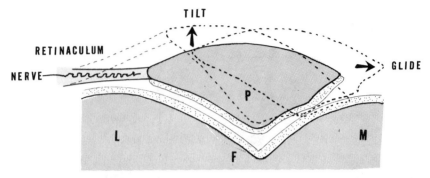

Figure 5–14. Retinacular attachment of the patella, allowing tilt and glide. The lateral retinaculum attaches to the lateral margin of the patella (P) seating it within the femoral (F), medial (M), and lateral (L) condyles. The retinaculum contains a sensory nerve.

The retinaculum should have significant flexibility to allow slight elevation (tilt) of the lateral margin of the patella and glide in the medial direction a distance of two quadrants of the patella. The cartilage is depicted as the shaded margins on the inferior border of the patella and the superior border of the femur.

If a lateral release fails to provide any benefit, displacement of the tibial tubercle may be needed (Fig. 5–17). This can be accomplished by medial transfer of the tubercle[28] or an anterior repositioning of the patellar tendon origin as in the Maquet[29] procedure. Either of these major surgical procedures must be undertaken with a great deal of trepidation. Every aspect of potential malalignment must be considered, such as varus, valgus, excessive patellar laxity, significant unresponsive quadriceps strengthening, tibial rotation, excessive Q angle, and so forth. Both procedures either

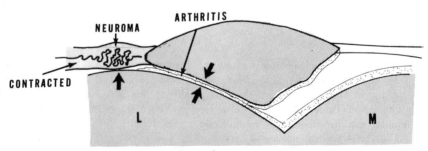

Figure 5–15. Lateral retinaculum contracture. As the lateral reticulum contracts (shortens), it thickens and entraps the nerve, creating a neuroma. The lateral facet of the patella becomes compressed (*arrows*) against the lateral femoral condyle (L) and causes compression and deterioration of the lateral facet articular surface, causing a degenerative "arthritis."

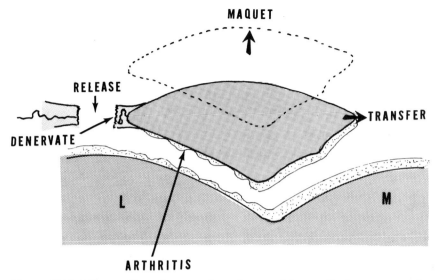

Figure 5–16. Effects of lateral retinacular release or Maquet displacement on the patella's position. A release of the lateral retinaculum allows the patella to glide medially (M) and simultaneously denervates the neuroma. The cartilage of the lateral facet of the patella is degenerated, as is the cartilage of the lateral femoral condyle (L). If a Maquet procedure[29] for transposing the tubercle attachment of the patella is performed, the patella ascends away (dotted lines indicating raised patella) from the femoral condyles (see Fig. 5–17).

medially transfer the patella into a more physiological position within the femoral condyles or elevate the patella "away" from the condyles.

Advancing the insertion of the vastus medialis muscle, releasing the lateral retinaculum, and lengthening the vastis lateralis are all involved in making the procedure extremely delicate.

Resurfacing the Patella

The degenerative changes in the surface of the patella and its movement on the femoral condyles have been assumed to be the cause of pain and impairment. Therefore, the procedure of shaving or debriding the patellar cartilage has been advocated. Regeneration of damaged cartilage is minimal, and even with replacement by fibrocartilage, the end results have been generally disappointing.

With the advent of arthroscopy, direct visualization of the damaged cartilage leads to a more precise, though limited, approach. The objective of shaving the patella is to remove loose material and leave an even surface. Some investigators claim that a clean, limited excision of the damaged

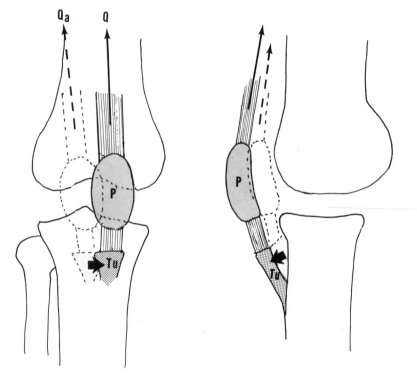

Figure 5–17. Procedures for relocating a malaligned patella. (*Left*) The figure demonstrates the medial translation of the tubercle (Tu) attachment of the infrapatellar tendon, which medially transposes the patella. The Q angle (Qa) is modified as the direction of the quadriceps (Q) is affected.

(*Right*) A lateral view of the Maquet procedure[29] in which the tibial tubercle (Tu) is anteriorly displaced, causing a separation of the patella (P) away from the femoral condyles. The direction of quadriceps pull is affected in the sagittal plane; however, the alignment is not affected (*arrows*).

patellar tissue permits recovery from the defect, but long-range follow-up studies are inconclusive. Prosthetic resurfacing is also in its infancy.[30,31]

Patellectomy

Patellectomy has been recommended for many years for severe patellar fractures, severe degenerative arthritis, rheumatoid arthritis, or painful recurrent subluxation of the patella.[32] Comminuted fracture was initially the primary indication for patellectomy because postreduction left an asymmetrical patella with a painful incongruency.

The rationale for patellectomy was that it removes the incongruous patella, and thus pain, "with no significant loss of quadriceps function."[33] As recently as 1989 the benefit of patellectomy for relief of pain with no functional loss of strength and function has been claimed,[34] but there are refuting claims[35] stating that patellectomy was considered functionally acceptable in only 5 percent of patients receiving this treatment, while 90 percent complained of residual "aching" and 60 percent complained of the knee "giving way."

Full clinical functional evaluation of postpatellectomy patients was unable to determine if there was any benefit with respect to protection of the underlying trochlea and distal femur by the patella from direct blows or compressive activities, such as ascending and descending stairs. The results were also inconclusive with regard to resumption of normal gait in walking and running, resumption of full athletic activities, knee stability, and cosmetic result.

Before advising patellectomy, the clinician must carefully evaluate the daily functional needs of the patient and weigh the limitations caused by the knee pathology in terms of pain acceptance and physical impairment. Replacement with a patella prosthesis is being explored and shows some promise. This technique may influence the choice of patellectomy in the future.

PLICA

The presence of an inflamed plica has been implicated as a cause of anterior knee pain. Plica, by definition, is a "fold," which in this case is a fold of the synovial lining of the knee joint. Numerous plications of any synovial tissue undoubtedly occur in a mobile joint in which there is redundancy of the synovial lining. Since the advent of arthroscopy, there have been many literature reports of plicae in the knee joint, and they have been implicated as a source of pain.

Three plicae have been described in the knee joint[36]: suprapatellar, infrapatellar, and medial patellar (Fig. 5–18). No lateral folds (plicae) have been described.

The suprapatellar plica is a synovial fold between the suprapatellar bursa and the knee joint proper. It is perforated into a "porta." The fold arises from the undersurface of the quadriceps tendon and attaches to the supermedial and superlateral wall of the joint. As the plica may be large and spacious with an opening, it may contain fragments of chondral debris. When thickened or inflamed, the fold (plica) may erode the superior aspect of the medial facet of the patella, across which the plica passes. It becomes horizontal on knee flexion (to 90°), at which point it may compress the femoral condylar surface.

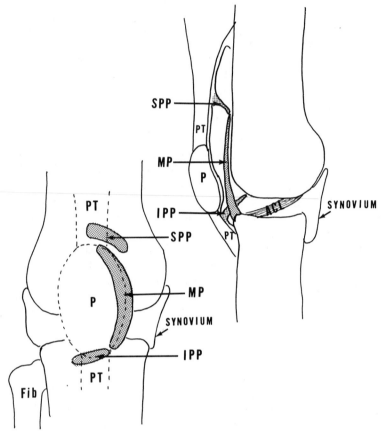

Figure 5–18. Plicae (synovial folds) of knee capsule. (*Left*) The figure shows the anterior view of the knee and the suprapatellar plica (SPP), the medial plica (MP), and the infrapatellar plica (IPP) in relation to the patella (P) and the patellar tendons (PTs). (*Right*) The figure depicts the lateral view of the same plicae and their relationship to the synovium and the anterior cruciate ligament (ACL).

The infrapatellar fold (plica) is located between the intercondylar notch and the infrapatellar fat pad. It has been termed the "ligamentum mucosum." Its clinical significance is questionable.

The medial patellar plica originates from the medial wall of the knee joint and runs downward in an oblique direction to insert with the synovium of the infrapatellar plica at the site of the infrapatellar fat pad. This medial plica may arise and be associated with the suprapatellar plica, or it may occur in the absence of the suprapatellar plica. The suprapatellar plica has also been called a "shelf," a "band," and "plica alaris elongata." Its presence in the knee joint varies from 18 to 55 percent.

As pathological entities, plicae can be considered sequelae to direct trauma of the knee joint, or secondary to hemarthrosis, regardless of the cause, or meniscal or anterior cruciate ligament injury. It could also be idiopathic.

When thickened, the medial plica may act as a taut bowstring impinging on the superior anteromedial portion of the medial femoral condyle, across which it allegedly stretches. The finding of medial patellar chondromalacia and femoral condyle arthrosis with a thickened plica is frequent, but the initial pathology remains unclear.

An inflamed plica should be considered most frequently as the diagnosis in the symptomatic knees of adolescent females. It accompanies numerous internal derangements of the knee, especially patellofemoral pathology, and is found on arthroscopic examination. The presence of an inflamed plica may be palpated and has been noted in magnetic resonance imaging (MRI) studies.

Patel[37] considers the medial patellar plica to be "a definitely pathological entity," but he also states that "a medial patellar plica exists 'normally' as a pleat . . . and should not necessarily be excised." "Although plicae are reported to be present in 20 percent of knees, the plica syndrome itself is uncommon. . . . The diagnosis is usually one of exclusion."[38] The significance of plica remains unknown.

PATELLAR DISLOCATION

While in motion, the patella remains within the confines of the femoral condyles because of the ligaments and tendons (Fig. 5–19), which are all related to the quadriceps mechanism. There is also a dependency on the patella's depth and contour and the condylar groove.

The inferior surface of the patella essentially presents two facets (medial and lateral) separated by a vertical ridge that is partially congruent with the grooves between the femoral condyle. Dislocation implies that the patella leaves this relationship and can be termed "luxation" (complete dislocation) or "subluxation" (partial dislocation). The latter has been alluded to repeatedly in previous discussions in this chapter.

Dislocation occurs for various reasons. Acute direct trauma can cause dislocation in an otherwise normal patellofemoral relationship. External injuries are predominantly caused by vehicular or athletic accidents. Dislocation may occur from lesser stress when there is femoral groove inadequacy from congenital dysplasia or from severe varus or valgus deformations (Fig. 5–20).

Acute dislocation as a result of direct trauma or congenital abnormality is self-evident. Recurrent dislocation poses significant clinical problems as to

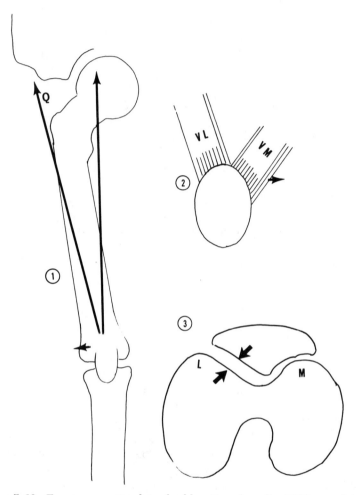

Figure 5–19. Forces preventing lateral subluxation of patella. (*1*) The quadriceps (Q) pull from the patella to anterior superior. The iliac crest is at an angle from the line of the femur; this angle is termed Q angle. (*2*) The vastus lateralis (VL) pulls the patella superiorly and laterally, while the vastus medialis (VM) neutralizes this by pulling the patella medially (*arrow*). (*3*) Superior view of patellofemoral joint showing the seating of the patella with the anterior femoral condyles. Lateral condyle (L) prevents lateral deviation; medial condyle (M) does not protrude to the same extent.

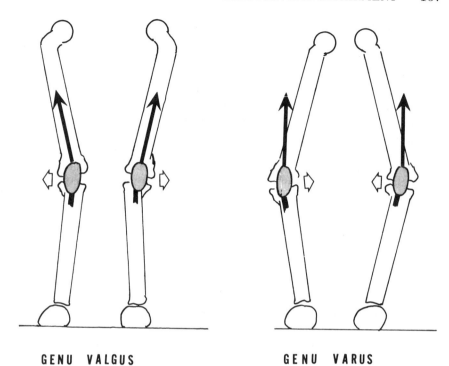

GENU VALGUS   **GENU VARUS**

Figure 5–20. Mechanism of patellar dislocation. There is lateral deviation of the patella in genu valgus and medial deviation in genu varus (*open arrows*); tibial or femoral rotation intensifies the stress.

diagnosis, acute treatment, and prevention of recurrence. An acute dislocation predisposes the knee to further episodes. The following are predisposing factors for recurrent dislocation (subluxation):

1. Marked genu valgum that laterally displaces the patella and improperly (laterally) aligns the extensor mechanism
2. Marked genu varus that medially displaces the patella
3. Excessive genu recurvatum, which relatively elongates the patellofemoral structures
4. An elongated infrapatellar tendon that results in a slack patellofemoral relation
5. A deficient vastus medialis muscle
6. Significant tibial external torsion
7. A shallow patellar groove of the femoral condyles
8. A shallow lateral femoral condyle
9. A laterally attached infrapatellar tendon on the tubercle
10. A deformed patella: congenital or posttraumatic

In a potential subluxing patella, there is a tendency for the knee to "buckle." The patient can actually fall. After a subluxation, pain and tenderness result and there may be effusion. Full extension of the knee may be impaired, but once the knee is extended, the patella returns to its normal seating if it was normal before the subluxation.

Examination should verify the underlying cause through meaningful x-rays, MRI, or CT scanning. There should also be a thorough, meaningful physical examination, which has already been discussed.

Treatment is obviously to correct the discovered pathology or deficiency. All conservative measures should be applied, but surgical procedures should be considered if these have failed or if there appears to be a surgically correctable basis for the dislocation. Modification of daily activities and/or athletic activities should be considered. An orthosis (patellar knee brace) may be successfully used while rehabilitation and healing occurs.

JUMPER'S KNEE

Patellar tendonitis was initially described by Blazina and associates[39] as a condition of young athletes who performed repeated jumping activities. The repetitive forces resulting from acceleration and deceleration in jumping activities caused overuse of the patellofemoral mechanism. It is veritably a traction overload, causing an overuse injury to the extensor mechanism. The pathology is in the bone tendon of the patellar mechanism, within the supra and infrapatellar ligaments and at the tubercle insertion. Because there is tearing of tendon fibrils, it is *not* a "tendonitis." There is no inflammation.

The most common site of pathology[40] is the inferior pole of the patella (65 percent), but there may be a pathology at the superior pole (25 percent) and at the tendinous attachment to the tubercle (10 percent) (Fig. 5–21). The collagen fibers of the tendon are torn, with resultant necrosis and repair by fibroblastic proliferation. Because the microtears do not necessarily initially result in significant pain, tenderness, or disability, the athlete continues with the stressful activity and causes further tissue injury.

The condition is progressive with recurrences in stages until perhaps irreversible pathology occurs. This results in chronic weakness of the patellar tendon. Continued traction on the patella may lead to an Osgood-Schlatter lesion (to be discussed later). If the athlete is sufficiently young so as not to have the epiphysis closed, a condition of epiphysitis, which is similar to Sinding-Larsen-Johansson disease (see Fig. 5–21), may result.[41] There may actually be an epiphyseal separation. The tendon may tear or there may be an avulsion fracture of the tibial tubercle, depending on the severity of the stress and the weakened condition of the injured tissues.

This condition must be recognized early and the joint "rested." It should also be treated conservatively to prevent the serious sequela that may permanently disable the athlete. The symptoms that lead to a diagnosis are local pain and tenderness noted after the physical activity (usually strenuous activities involving the knee, such as repeated forceful jumping). After the onset of activities the pain may decrease or disappear after "warm up" only to recur after completion of the athletic activity. If there is progression of the lesion, the pain may start with the activity, remain throughout the activity, and persist after rest.

At first the pain is a dull ache that may become sharper and more of a "pain." The pain now occurs not only after athletic activities but after ascending or descending stairs, doing deep knee bends or squats, arising from a chair after prolonged sitting, and even after prolonged walking. The patient may complain of the knee "giving out" or "being weak." There may develop a reluctance to participate in physical activities.

Effusion is rare and when present indicates the possibility of *other* knee pathology with or without tubercle tendon pathology. On examination there is palpable tenderness of the poles of the tendon, the tendon itself, or the superior aspect of the tubercle. This palpation should be done with the knee

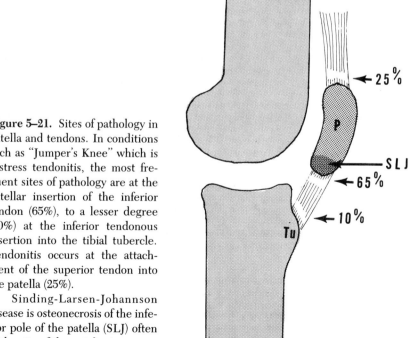

Figure 5–21. Sites of pathology in patella and tendons. In conditions such as "Jumper's Knee" which is a stress tendonitis, the most frequent sites of pathology are at the patellar insertion of the inferior tendon (65%), to a lesser degree (10%) at the inferior tendonous insertion into the tibial tubercle. Tendonitis occurs at the attachment of the superior tendon into the patella (25%).

Sinding-Larsen-Johannson disease is osteonecrosis of the inferior pole of the patella (SLJ) often at the site of the epiphysis.

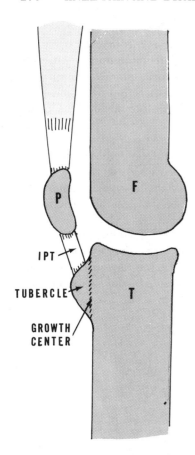

Figure 5–22. Osgood-Schlatter disease. The lateral view of the knee joint (F, femur; T, tibia; and P, patella) depicts the attachment of the infrapatellar tensor (IPT) to the tibial tubercle. Before maturation and when the tubercle growth center is fused, a traction injury can separate the two adjacent bones (tubercle and tibia). This separation has been called Osgood-Schlatter disease.

relaxed in the fully extended position. X-ray findings of translucency have been described. In young people the x-ray studies may reveal fragmentation of the inferior pole of the patella consistent with Sinding-Larsen-Johannson disease. More recently bone scanning has been described as diagnostic when done early in the disease process.[42]

The patellar tubercle should always be examined carefully to rule out an Osgood-Schlatter lesion (Fig. 5–22), which is a traction epiphysitis of the tibial tubercle. If there is progression of the pathology, the dreaded result is a tear of the tendon. The tear may be palpable with one patella riding higher than the other. Weakness of quadriceps contraction against resistance is noted, and knee extension may be impossible. X-ray verification reveals the patella riding higher than the one on the contralateral side, verifying the existence of the patellar tendon lesion.

When a previously recurrent injury is stressed and there is residual immature epiphyseal closure, avulsion of the patellar tubercle may result[43] (Fig. 5–23).

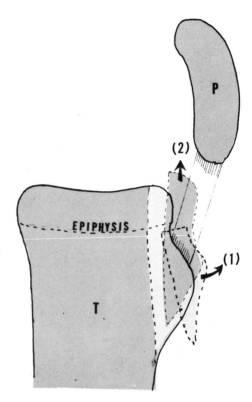

Figure 5–23. Avulsion fractures of the tibial tubercle. Most avulsion fractures of the tibial tubercle are the results of athletic injuries to adolescent individuals who may still have incompletely closed epiphyses. The tubercle can be avulsed anteriorly (1), or it can be elevated in a sagittal plane (2). The latter deforms the tibial plateau.

Sinding-Larsen-Johannson disease is essentially a traction epiphysitis of the inferior pole of the patella. The epiphysis becomes fragmented and an avascular necrosis ensues. Ultimately fibrous tissue and then ossification appear. The patella may be deformed and the patellar tendon rendered inadequate.

Osgood-Schlatter Disease

The possibility of an Osgood-Schlatter syndrome (Fig. 5–24) must also be considered since this is a variant of the epiphysial traction separation. The epiphysis in this case is that of the tibial tubercle to which is attached the infrapatellar tendon. This syndrome, as is the Sinding-Larsen-Johansson syndrome, is ultimately diagnosed radiologically, but it must be suspected clinically. The Sinding-Larsen-Johansson syndrome presents tenderness over the inferior aspect of the patella, whereas the Osgood-Schlatter syndrome presents tenderness over the tibial tubercle.

Treatment of Osgood-Schlatter disease consists of avoiding activities that impose traction on the patellotubercle site and avoiding direct pressure,

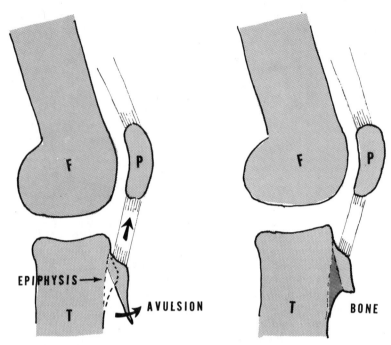

Figure 5–24. Osgood-Schlatter lesion. After an avulsion of the patellar tubercle at the epiphyseal line there is fibrotic healing with ultimate ossification (shown as bone in the right illustration). The bony deformed tubercle remains firmly attached to the infrapatellar tendon but changes slightly the alignment of the patellar pull. It is also a hindrance to kneeling.

as in kneeling. In severe cases a cylindrical cast may be applied for several months during which quadriceps exercises within the cast *must* be initiated. Surgical repair such as multiple drillings, bone grafting, or tendon splinting has been advocated.

Treatment of Sinding-Larsen-Johannson disease consists of curtailing and preferably avoiding stressful activities. Casting may be indicated if the condition is severe, but this is fraught with the danger of quadriceps atrophy and limitation of the joint's range of motion.

Progression of any pathology of the patellar-tendon-tubercle complex may lead to complete separation of the infrapatellar tendon, its attachment to the tubercle, or attachment of the tubercle to the tibia (see Fig. 5–23). An avulsion "fracture" of the tubercle occurs. This becomes evident when knee extension failure occurs in normal daily activities and athletic activities. Weakness becomes apparent when the knee "gives out" because full extension is no longer possible. Since deep knee bends are impossible, getting up from a chair and ascending and descending stairs are impaired. On testing, full knee extension is limited and not possible against any resistance.

The patella rides higher than the contralateral side on examination. This acquired "alta" patellar position can be identified on lateral x-ray views. Why these pathological syndromes occur is conjectural. The excessive force of the athletic activity and excessive exposure of the joint "overuse" are claimed, but other factors have been explored. Patella alta, hypermobility of the patella, significant genu varus or valgum, and tibial torsion have all been considered a prerequisite,[44] but no common denominator has emerged.

The surface of the terrain on which the sport is performed appears the best predictor of pathology. A hard surface such as concrete is commonly cited. The frequency and duration of the athletic activity have also been implicated. It can be assumed that the jumper's knee can occur in any athlete with as yet immature epiphysial closure.

Treatment of Jumper's Knee

Early recognition of significant pathological changes in the anterior knee patellar-tibial-tubercle complex is mandatory. Since the condition occurs mostly in highly motivated, competitive athletes and initially does not impair function but merely presents discomfort, curtailing or even modifying athletic activities is a difficult solution.

In the early stage, where any discomfort after activity subsides with activity yet recurs immediately after the activity, treatment may consist of:

1. Resting the part. This means:
   a. Discontinuing the athletic activity for several months.
   b. Avoiding deep knee bends, squats, and ascending and descending stairs.
2. Local application of ice for 20-minute periods at least four times daily.
3. Oral anti-inflammatory medication. Local injection of steroid is to be avoided since there is evidence that the tendinous collagen may be adversely affected by local injection of steroids.[45]
4. Avoidance of splinting or casting since this initiates early quadriceps weakness and atrophy.
5. "Warm up exercises" should be undertaken before resuming the activities. These include:
   a. Gentle, progressive hamstring and heel cord stretching.
   b. Gentle, progressive isometric quadriceps exercises.
   c. Progressive to active quadriceps isotonic exercises.
6. Local application of heat to the anterior knee prior to athletic activity.
7. Evaluation of pronation and genu valgum or varus with appropriate orthosis. An elastic knee orthosis has been advocated[46] as being beneficial and is worth trying on resumption of athletic activity.
8. Use of a well-cushioned athletic shoe with proper inserts.

The discovery of the potential for jumper's knee and its progression demands education of the athlete as to the need for immediately reporting the recurrence of symptoms and even the possibility that discontinuance of further athletic participation may be required. The athletic coach and parents must be included in the care of the athlete.

If there is recurrence, and especially if there is progression of the symptoms* and reluctance of the athlete to discontinue his or her participation, surgical intervention may be indicated. The exact surgical procedure is based on the surgeon's experience since there is, as yet, no standard accepted procedure. The procedure recommended by Colosimo and Bassett[47] addresses the site and type of pathology within the tendon. The pathological histological findings are myxomatous changes, disruption of collagen fiber alignment, and replacement with fibrocartilaginous tissue. As each layer of the patellar tendon is examined, the pathological tissue is debrided and the contiguous tissues are reapproached and sutured. Rehabilitation is begun immediately after surgery with quadriceps exercises begun to the tolerance of the patient. Return to athletic activities has been achieved within 6 months.

OSTEOCHONDRITIS DISSECANS

In this painful knee condition there is fragmentation of articular cartilage with a varying degree of inclusion of some subchondral bone (Fig. 5–25). The fragment may remain in situ or completely avulse from the remaining bone and become a foreign body within the joint. This condition occurs in children, predominantly in males.

The onset is usually insidious with the pain described as aching and poorly localized. Stiffness is often claimed. When the dissecans presents a loose joint body, the knee may "lock" and "give out."

The etiological factors have been considered to be:

1. Direct trauma to the inner aspect of the femur by the opposing tibial tuberosity. This is especially possible if the joint has been narrowed by a torn cartilage in a patient with severe valgus or varus.

2. Heredity.

3. Local circumscribed circulatory obstruction from a thrombus or an embolus. This is an unlikely explanation since the condition is frequently bilateral and multiple.

4. Endocrine imbalance. This is conjectural since the precise endocrine imbalance has yet to be ascertained.

---

*Even after a period of rest of 3 to 6 months, symptoms frequently reoccur when athletic activities are resumed.[47]

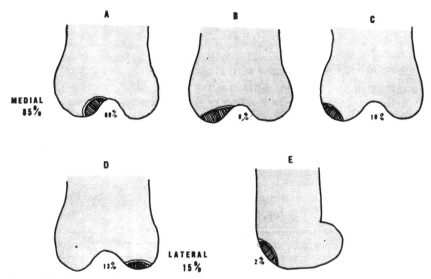

Figure 5–25. Sites of osteochondritis dissecans of the knee. *(Top)* Most (85 percent) occur on the medial femoral condyle; *(A)* classical with 69 percent on the lateral border of the medial condyle; *(B)* extended classical with 6 percent; *(C)* an inferocentral site with 10 percent. *(Bottom)* 15 percent occur on the lateral condyle; *(D)* inferocentral with 13 percent; *(E)* an anterior site with 2 percent.

5. Anomaly of ossification if the condition occurs before the age of 10. In juvenile osteochondritis (age 15) and adult osteochondritis these factors are not considered significant.

Osteochondritis dissecans of the patella is a rare condition but one that should be entertained in a young athletic individual who complains of anterior knee pain. Only 70 cases have been reported in the literature.[48] It has led to the conviction that repeated microtrauma, especially shear force, is a causative factor.[49] A good example is found in the report about a young competitive fencer.[48] Fencing requires that the back leg be held in a slightly flexed position while the lower leg is externally rotated. The forward leg receives multiple thrusts. The repeated shear forces on the bent knee caused the observed condition.

Physical findings are sparse and are not at all indicative of what causes the symptoms. There may be quadriceps atrophy if the condition has been symptomatic and caused avoidance of activity. There may be tenderness over the femoral condyle region and the loose body may be palpable.

Diagnosis is made by x-ray verification and localization and by severity of pain. Numerous views of the knee may be required for confirmation (see Fig. 5–26).

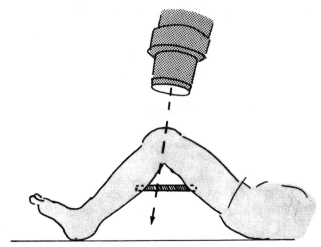

Figure 5–26. An x-ray skyline view for visualizing the femoral condyles.

The routine multiple-view x-rays, especially the tangential patellar projection, reveal the defect; however, more recent MRI studies clearly reveal not only the defect but also the attachment of the osteochondral fragment by a soft tissue "hinge."

Treatment in very young children consists of immobilization in a cylindrical cast. Surgical removal of the fragment is indicated if there is a loose joint body of significant size with encroachment on the tibiofemoral condylar cartilage. Severity and persistence of symptoms are also an indication for surgery, especially if there is failure of compliance with long periods of inactivity. Some have advocated nailing the fragment back into its original bed.[50–52] Lesions greater than 20 mm in diameter lead to a poor prognosis, as does the lack of surrounding normal supporting cartilage.[53]

REFERENCES

1. Radin, EL: Anterior knee pain, the need for a specific diagnosis: Stop calling it chondromalacia! Orthop Rev 14:128, 1985.
2. Radin, EL: A rational approach to the treatment of patellofemoral pain. Clin Orthop Rel Res 144:107, 1979.
3. Haxton, R: The function of the patella and the effects of its excision. Surg Gynecol Obstet 80:389, 1945.
4. Bruce, J and Walmsley, R: Excision of the patella: Some experimental and anatomical observations. J Bone Joint Surg 24:311, 1942.
5. Scott, JC: Fractures of the patella. J Bone Joint Surg 31B:76, 1949.
6. Sutton, FS, Jr, et al: The effect of patellectomy on knee function. J Bone Joint Surg 58A:537, 1976.
7. Gardner, E: The innervation of the knee joint. Anat Rec 101:109, 1948.

8. Cailliet, R: Mechanics of Joints, Arthritis and Physical Medicine, Vol 11. Waverly Press, Baltimore, 1969.

9. Chrisman, OD, Ladenbauer-Bellis, IM, and Panjabi, M: The relationship of mechanical trauma and early reactions of osteoarthritic cartilage. Clin Orthop 161:265, 1981.

10. Mankin, HJ: The reaction of articular cartilage to injury and osteoarthritis: Medical progress. New Engl J Med 291:1285, 1974.

11. Collins, DH and McElliot, TF: Sulphate uptake by chondrocytes in relation to histological changes in osteoarthritic human articular cartilage. Ann Rheum Dis 19:318, 1960.

12. Chrisman, OD, Ladenbauer-Bellis, IM, and Fulkerson, JP: The osteoarthritic cascade and associated drug actions. Seminars Arthr Rheum (Suppl) 11:145, 1981.

13. Thomas, CL (ed): Taber's Cyclopedic Medical Dictionary, ed 15. FA Davis, Philadelphia, 1985, p 281.

14. Chrisman, OD, Fessel, JM, and Southwick, WO: Experimental production of synovitis and marginal articular exostosis in knee joints of dogs. Yale J Biol Med 37:409, 1965.

15. Karlson, S: Chondromalacia patella. Acta Chir Scand 83:347, 1939.

16. Kulowski, J: Chondromalacia of the patella, fissural cartilage degeneration: Traumatic chondropathy. Report of three cases. JAMA 100:1837, 1933.

17. Wiles, P, Andrews, PS, and Devas, MB: Chondromalacia of the patella. J Bone Joint Surg 38B:95, 1956.

18. Goodfellow, J, Hungerford, DS, and Woods, C: Patellofemoral joint mechanics and pathology, 2: Chondromalacia patellae. J Bone Joint Surg 58B:291, 1976.

19. Laurin, CA, et al: The tangential x-ray investigation of the patellofemoral joint. X-ray technique, diagnostic criteria and their interpretation. Clin Orthop 144:16, 1979.

20. Merchant, AC: Isolated patellofemoral arthritis: Its significance and treatment. Cont Orthop 3:1015, 1981.

21. Insall, J: Chondromalacia patellae: Patellar malalignment syndrome. Orthop Clin North Amer 10:117, 1979.

22. Schuter, SF, Ramsby, GR, and Fulkerson, JP: Computed tomographic classification of patellofemoral pain patients. Orthop Clinics N Amer 17:235, 1986.

23. Dye, S, et al: Assessing patellar scintigraphic activity—a new quantitative method. Orthop Transactions 9:459, 1985.

24. DeHaven, KE, Dolan, WA, and Mayer, PJ: Chondromalacia patellae in athletes: Clinical presentation and conservative management. Amer J Sports Med 7:5, 1979.

25. Stougard, J: Chondromalacia of the patella: Physical signs in relation to operative findings. Acta Orthop Scan 46:685, 1975.

26. Cailliet, R: Low Back Pain, ed 4. FA Davis, Philadelphia, 1988.

27. Kolowich, PA, et al: Lateral release of the patella: Indications and contraindications. Amer J Sports Med 18:359, 1990.

28. Cox, JS: Evaluation of the Roux-Elmslie-Trillat procedure for knee extensor realignment. Amer J Sports Med 10:303, 1982.

29. Maquet, PGJ: Biomechanics of the knee. Springer-Verlag, New York, 1976.

30. Insall, JN, Tria, AJ, and Aglietti, P: Resurfacing of the patella. J Bone Joint Surg 62A:933, 1980.

31. Worrell, RV: Prosthetic resurfacing of the patella. Clin Orthop 144:91, 1979.

32. Cohn, BNE: Total and partial patellectomy: An experimental study. Surg Gynecol Obstet 79:526, 1944.

33. Brooke, R: The treatment of fractured patella by excision: A study of morphology and function. Brit J Surg 24:733, 1937.

34. Jensen, DB: Patellectomy for chondromalacia. Acta Orthop Scand 60:17, 1989.

35. Scott, JC: Fractures of the patella. J Bone Joint Surg 31B:76, 1949.

36. Patel D: Arthroscopy of the plica-synovial folds and their significance. Amer J Sports Med 6:217, 1978.

37. Patel, D: Plica as a cause of anterior knee pain. Orthop Clinics N Amer 17:273, 1986.

38. Kinnard, P and Levesque, RY: The plica syndrome: A syndrome controversy. Clin Orthop 183:141, 1984.
39. Blazina, ME, et al: Jumper's knee. Orthop Clin N Amer 4:665, 1973.
40. Ferretti, A, et al: The natural history of jumper's knee. Int Orthop (SICOT) 8:239, 1985.
41. Medlar, RC and Lyne, ED: Sinding-Larsen-Johannson disease. J Bone Joint Surg 60A:1113, 1978.
42. Kahn, D and Wilson, M: Bone scintigraphic findings in patellar tendinitis. J Nuc Med 28:1768, 1987.
43. Ogden, JA, Tross, PB, and Murphy, MJ: Fracture of the tibial tuberosity in adolescents. J Bone Joint Surg 62A:205, 1980.
44. Mariani, PP, Puddu, G, and Ferretti, A: Jumper's knee. Ital J Orthop Traumatol 4:85, 1978.
45. Martens, M, et al: Patellar tendinitis: Pathology and results of treatment. Acta Orthop Scand 53:445, 1982.
46. Palumbo, PM: Dynamic patellar brace: A new orthosis in the management of patellofemoral disorders—a preliminary report. Amer J Sports Med 9:45, 1981.
47. Colosimo, AJ and Bassett, FH: Jumper's knee, diagnosis and treatment: A review paper. Othop Review 29:139, 1990.
48. Desaii, S, et al: Osteochondritis dissecans of the patella. J Bone Joint Surg 69B:320, 1987.
49. Gray, WJ and Bassett, FH: Osteochondritis dissecans of the patella in a competitive fencer. Orthopedic Review 19(1):96, 1990.
50. Wiberg, G: Spontaneous healing of osteochondritis dissecans in the knee joint. Acta Orthop Scand 12:319, 1941.
51. Aichroth, P: Osteochondritis dissecans of the knee. J Bone Joint Surg 53B:440, 1971.
52. Smillie, IS: Osteochondritis dissecans of the knee. Amer J Orthop 6:236, 1964.
53. Edwards, DH and Bently, G: Osteochondritis dissecans patellae. J Bone Joint Surg 59B:58, 1977.

CHAPTER 6
Arthritides Affecting the Knee

MONOARTICULAR ARTHRITIS

The knee can be involved in a monoarticular arthritic inflammation; that is, it can be the only joint of the body involved. It may have restricted joint motion, swelling, redness, and heat, all indicating an intra-articular inflammation. The clinician must determine that the knee is the only joint involved. The differential diagnosis is between an infection and an inflammation, which requires a synovial aspiration (Fig. 6–1). A bacterial culture and a blood cell determination must follow.

An elevated leukocyte count with a high percentage of polymorphonuclear cells suggests infection. The presence of crystals suggests a gouty arthritis. A low serum complement is suggestive of rheumatoid arthritis or lupus, whereas an elevated serum complement suggests Reiter's syndrome. The trauma that caused the monoarticular effusion must be determined from a careful history or by direct observation.

The treatment and management of one of these specific monoarticular diseases depend on the precise diagnosis. Management of the residual damage to the joint also depends on the extent and type of damage to the cartilage, synovium, capsule, and tendons.

POLYARTICULAR ARTHRITIS

When there is evidence that the inflamed and swollen knee is only one of many affected joints, a differential diagnosis must be made. These vary from rheumatoid arthritis (RA) or its variants, lupus erythematosus, polyarthritis, sarcoid, psoriasis, or ochronosis. "Only a careful analysis of the synovial fluid changes, blood count, biopsy, physical findings, etc. will

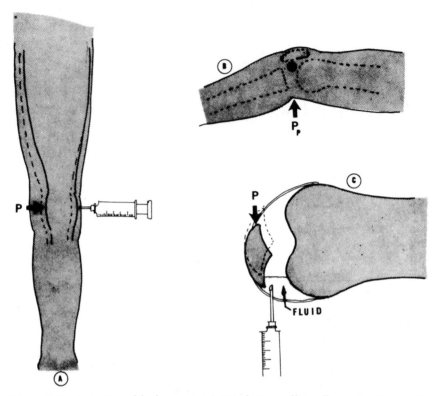

Figure 6–1. Aspiration of the knee joint. (A) Technique of laterally moving the patella (P) to increase the injectable space between the patella and the femoral condyle. (B) Lateral view, site of injection (*black dot*) and popliteal space pressure (P_p) to bring fluid to needle tip. (C) With lateral position, the fluid gravitates to permit easier aspiration.

ultimately result in a specific diagnosis which will lead to specific treatment."[1]

RHEUMATOID ARTHRITIS

Rheumatoid arthritis is a systemic disease, an inflammatory disorder of connective tissue with primary involvement of synovial membranes. There are many parenchymal tissues involved, such as small arteries, tendons, and their sheaths, ligaments, and the joint capsules. The structures of the knee that become involved are the capsular tissues and the synovium of the cartilage as shown in Figure 6–2.

The diagnosis of rheumatoid arthritis is made on clinical grounds and is confirmed by laboratory tests. The diagnostic criteria have been postulated

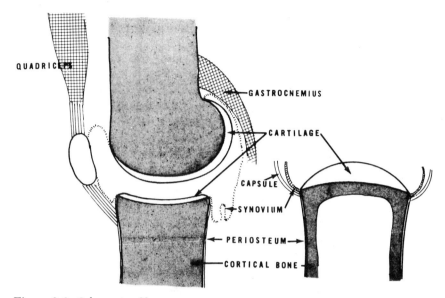

Figure 6–2. Schematic of knee joint structures. *(Left)* Structures forming the joint; *(Right)* Graphic illustration of the relationship of the capsule and the synovial membrane to the cartilaginous-cortical union.

by the American Rheumatism Association. They include (1) morning stiffness, (2) pain on joint motion, (3) symmetrical swelling of joints, (4) subcutaneous nodules, (5) typical changes seen on x-ray film, and (6) a positive test for rheumatoid factor.

Pathophysiology

Rheumatoid inflammation begins with hyperemic congestion, edema, and cellular infiltration by plasma cells and lymphocytes, with the latter being prominent. However, in the acute phase, there may be a large proportion of polymorphs present. In the early phase of the disease, the joint cartilage surface becomes covered with fibrinoid material, while fibroblasts and capillaries invade the synovial tissue. This latter invasion thickens the underlying synovial tissue. Simultaneously the synovial fluid reflects the inflammatory reaction. The surrounding joint capsule, contiguous tendons, and ligaments also undergo inflammatory reactions that remain, to this date, nonspecific in their pathophysiology.

As the process continues, marginal erosions in the subchondral bone occur. A pannus appears on the cartilage, and the cartilage undergoes degenerative changes (Fig. 6–3). Pannus is an apron of granular vascular tissue that consists of proliferating fibroblasts, collagen fibers, small blood

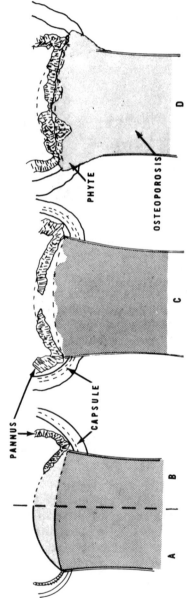

Figure 6–3. Progressive stages of rheumatoid disease of a joint. (*A*) The normal half of a joint. (*B*) Early thickening of the synovium, caused by edema, congestion, and invasion of fibroblasts and capillaries. The thickened synovium is termed pannus and gradually covers the cartilage. The capsule thickens. (*C*) Pannus gradually invades and replaces the cartilage, and the subchondral bone undergoes erosion. (*D*) Advanced stage of the disease with loss of cartilage replaced by fibrous pannus, erosion of the subchondral bone, osteophyte (marginal) formation, and osteoporosis of the cortex. Only one bone that forms the joint has been shown, but the same condition is occurring simultaneously in all the bones of the joint.

vessels, and numerous varied inflammatory blood cells. Whereas originally it was believed that the pannus preceded and was responsible for the ultimate cartilage damage, it now appears that the pannus is the result of cartilage damage. Joints that have been studied during the early weeks of rheumatoid arthritis have revealed early degenerative changes along with depletion of cartilage matrix and, as yet, *no* pannus formation. It has been postulated that the pannus does not *invade* the cartilage but rather is formed by conversion of cartilage into fibrous tissue through the metamorphosis of chondrocytes into fibroblasts. The exact mechanism and cause of the initial cartilage destruction remain unknown. The breakdown of the cartilage is probably related to an alteration in the blood immune system.

The interface between the pannus and the cartilage has been found to be crossed by fine collagen fibers, which may indicate that the pannus is not a destructive agent but rather is engaged in repairing the damaged cartilage with nonspecific fibrous tissue. Studies[2] indicate that the granular tissue that replaces the damaged cartilage is *not* a direct extension of synovium but rather is an invasion from the subchondral vascular spaces and from the marrow through the subchondral plate (Fig. 6–4). Pannus formation is thus considered to be a late phenomenon that follows the subchondral invasion. Synovial disease may well initiate the process with all subsequent reactions being secondary.

Normal cartilage contains water, collagen, and a protein polysaccharide matrix. It is thought that chondrocytes secrete the matrix that provides the

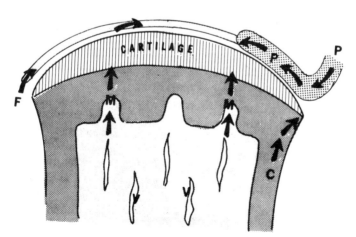

Figure 6–4. Schematic route of articular disease. The fibrinoid film (F) covers the cartilage and ultimately undergoes organization. Pannus (P), which is inflamed synovium that contains fibroblasts and capillaries, has fine collagen fibers connecting to the cartilage. Marrow (M) and cortex (C) invasion of osteoclasts penetrates the subcortical bone plate to invade the cartilage and ultimately destroy it from within. V = deep blood vessels.

rigidity and elasticity of the cartilage. The matrix is traversed by interwoven fibrils that reinforce the cartilage. The matrix has a limited life span and must constantly be renewed by the chondrocytes. Rheumatoid arthritis may arise from impairment of chondrocyte function (Fig. 6–5).

Lysosomes, which allegedly are capable of degrading cartilage, are membrane-bound organelles that contain proteinases, carbohydrases, and lipases. These enzymes are capable of hydrolyzing proteins, carbohydrates, and lipids, respectively. In rheumatoid arthritis a "factor" is released that possibly ruptures the lysosomal membrane and releases the enzymes that subsequently attack the chondrocytes. This factor is thought to be an immunoglobulin involved in an autoimmune response. In rheumatoid arthritis a protein called *fibrin* is also released; this protein lines the cartilage and denies it the necessary nutrients.

In summary, rheumatoid arthritis is currently believed to be an

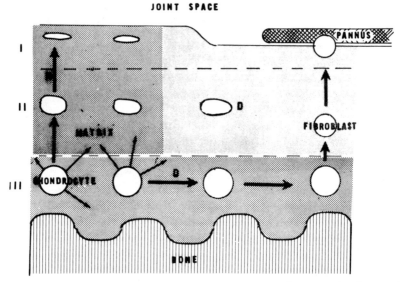

Figure 6–5. Schematic of theory of cartilage degradation in rheumatoid arthritis. The chondrocytes, located in the basal layers (III), secrete the matrix (primarily water, collagen, and protein polysaccharides). As the chondrocyte ages, it migrates (*arrows*) toward the joint space (N). As degradation (D) occurs (cause unknown), the intermediate zone (II) loses metachromatic mucopolysaccharide (stains alkaline) and (I) is the superficial layer that comprises dessicated endothelial cells. A theory is expounded which claims that some chondrocytes become fibroblasts that migrate peripherally to form the pannus. The pannus consists of vascular granulating tissue, proliferating fibroblasts, inflammatory cells, and collagen fibers. The chondrocytes may begin degradation when they are attacked by enzymes liberated from the lysosomes, which in turn were damaged by an infectious agent, for example, a virus or bacteria.

autoimmune antibody reaction that attacks the lysosomal capsule and releases its lytic enzymes. The evidence[3] that there is an immune process in RA is:

1. Lymphoid cell infiltration of the synovium
2. Synthesis of IgG and a rheumatoid factor (RF) by plasma cells
3. Decreased complement component in the synovia
4. Presence of both IgG and IgM in the cells of the synovial lining, leukocytes, and synovial fluid

Subsequently there is synovial inflammation with thickening and reduction of an abnormal synovial fluid, which may also contain abnormal substrates. This capsular thickening subsequent to synovitis accompanies the destruction of the articular cartilage, and thus the joint mechanism becomes gradually impaired.

Marginal osteophytes organize because of the changes occurring at the capsular bone junction (see Fig. 6–3). The progression of joint changes in RA is either a fibrous ankylosis or progressive degenerative osteoarthrosis.

Treatment

In planning a treatment program for the patient with rheumatoid arthritis, the physician should consider the status of the joint's function. This is influenced by (1) the duration of the disease and its severity, (2) age, sex, occupation, and family responsibilities of the patient and (3) the results of any previous treatment.

The disease usually follows the sequence of pathological events (Fig. 6–6) shown below:

Phase I: Soft tissue involvement. This is primarily synovial hyperemia with some joint effusion. The knee is swollen, hot, and tender. The capsule is swollen, and the surrounding ligaments are stretched, inflamed, and tender. At this stage, x-ray films merely reveal soft tissue swelling with normal joint space features. A bone scan and magnetic resonance imaging (MRI) would reveal inflammation.

Phase II: This is the stage when synovitis is accompanied by the formation of pannus. There is some underlying bone destruction that becomes apparent on x-ray studies. At this stage arthroscopy would reveal the synovitis and the presence of pannus. MRI studies would reveal the status of the ligament and cartilage damage.

Phase III: In this stage there is cartilage destruction and subchondral bone erosion with narrowing of the joint space. Clinically there is instability of the joint. The soft tissue swelling has diminished or disappeared, and the

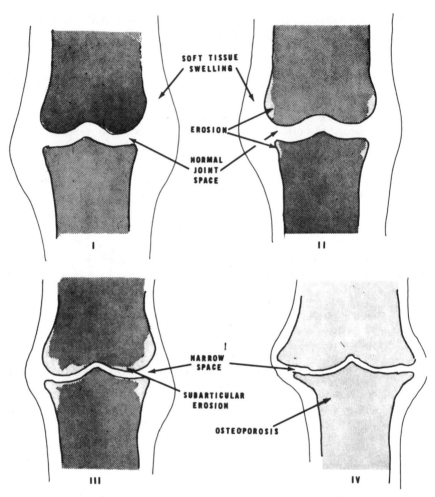

Figure 6–6. Changes in rheumatoid arthritis seen by x-ray study. (*Phase I*) Early signs reveal soft tissue swelling with a normal joint space. Occasionally, the swelling may separate the involved joint. (*Phase II*) As the disease progresses, some erosion is noted at the lateral margins where the collateral ligaments attach. (*Phase III*) The erosion spreads centrally to the subchondral region, and the joint space narrows. (*Phase IV*) The joint space becomes occluded as the cartilage completely disappears and bone opposes bone; the capsule is not fibrotic and not swollen (effused). There are bilateral osteophytes.

periarticular swelling is more like an induration because of the fibrous reaction.

Phase IV: The degree of cartilage destruction and the decalcification of the bone are now apparent on routine x-ray films. Clinically there is marked joint laxity, which also implies ligamentous destruction and painful "grating" during passive and active joint motion, which is limited in all ranges. Osteophytosis of the marginal borders is noted on routine x-ray studies.

There is currently no cure for rheumatoid arthritis, but there are agents that temporarily diminish the articular symptoms and the severity of joint destruction. These agents also permit conservative physical therapy.

Aspirin remains the mainstay of systemic therapy, and the frequent daily doses should be monitored to achieve the optimum therapeutic dosage with minimal side effects. The mechanism of action of aspirin has been well documented and will not be discussed here. All aspirin-type drugs, including nonsteroidal anti-inflammatory drugs (NSAIDs), are inhibitors of prostaglandin synthesis. In severe chronic, active rheumatoid arthritis, the use of cryotherapy (gold) remains a valid procedure and needs to be implemented by a qualified experienced physician.

Periods of rest during the day are of value since this is a systematic disease. Prolonged and excessive rest, however, is to be avoided since it can result in further muscular weakness, atrophy, joint contracture, and systemic debility.

Local Joint Therapeutic Management. Unlike other knee joint impairments that have been listed elsewhere in this text, the principles of rest, and splinting followed by passive and active motion need clarification. In RA, the definition of excessive rest and immobilization varies in relationship to other traumatic or degenerative conditions of the knee.

The rheumatoid arthritic knee is of concern. In an acute, active, inflammatory condition, repetitive motion is to be avoided since it creates undesirable joint stress and enhances inflammation. It is desirable to rest the part until the medical therapeutic agents begin to have an effect. The joint can be rested during the frequent periods of total rest required in treating the systemic RA condition.

Splinting of the knee in a physiological position (Fig. 6–7) is desirable, providing it is associated with other means of rehabilitation to prevent

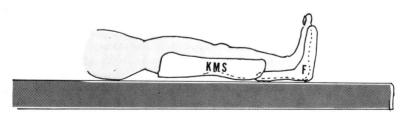

Figure 6–7. Posterior molded knee splint. The patient lies in a supine position and has the knee maintained in the fully extended position by a posterior molded splint (KMS). The foot and ankle can be held in a right angle position by a posterior molded foot-ankle splint (F). The mattress is firm.

atrophy, weakness (especially of the quadriceps), and contracture of the joint capsule. A firm bed mattress is also desirable. During sleep the patient should avoid knee flexion by judicious use of pillows. The knee must be kept fully extended. Unfortunately, the knee feels slightly less painful at a few degrees of flexion, but this position must be avoided and the patient must be informed about the undesirable sequelae. The frequently assumed prone position prevents hip flexion contracture, which can ultimately have an adverse mechanical effect on the knee when erect posture and ambulation are resumed.

Local modalities afford pain relief and conceivably minimize production of nociceptors. Ice packs, ice cubes within a plastic container, are applied for 20 minutes several times daily and are beneficial because they relieve pain, decrease edema, minimize inflammation, and decrease the discomfort of passive and isometric exercise. The application of local heat using a moist compress is beneficial and is often better tolerated than an ice pack. Alternating ice packs and heat packs have many advocates (hot-cold contrast). Ultrasound may have physiological advantages, but the need to transport a patient to a center to receive this treatment usually negates its value.

To maintain quadriceps muscular function, the patient should begin isometric contractions *as early as they can be tolerated.* Slow, gradual, sustained quadriceps contraction should be done on a schedule, such as a specific number of contractions every one-half hour to every hour (for example, 5 to 10 isometric contractions per hour). Each session should be preceded by ice packs and followed by hot, moist compresses.

As soon as they are tolerated by the patient, isotonic exercises should be instituted and encouraged by the therapist. At first the patient is instructed to isotonically contract the quadriceps with the knee slightly flexed (5° to 10°) and gradually to increase the isotonic contractions from full extension to 90° flexion and then the reverse. Resistance can, and should be, added gradually. Loss of knee extension and quadriceps strength is the major functional loss of rheumatoid arthritic patients who have knee joint involvement.

Passive range of motion has value but must be carefully and judiciously applied. An excessive range of motion is to be avoided during the acute inflammatory phase because the soft tissues are subject to deformation, and the motion can lead to minor subluxation and postacute phase instability. Placing the knee through flexion and extension is desirable and must be performed at least several times daily. At first during severe acute inflammation passive exercises that include three to four ranges of motion done twice daily may be all that is tolerable and desirable. As the inflammation subsides, the frequency and duration of the exercises can be gradually increased.

The medial collateral ligaments have been shown to be adversely affected in RA, and stressing or stretching of the ligaments while positioning the knee or performing passive exercises must be assiduously avoided. The foot and ankle joint must not be allowed to develop flexion contracture. While in the posterior molded knee splint, the ankle must also be maintained at 90° dorsiflexion. An equinus deformity of the foot and ankle joint hinders normal gait[4] and places undue stress on the knee during ambulation (see Chap. 9).

When the patient is able to resume walking, the knee should be protected by the use of crutches and or a walker. A soft knee splint that keeps the knee in full extension is also indicated initially.

Surgical Intervention. If the patient still suffers from active synovitis after a reasonable period (usually estimated as 6 months, but it is variable) of conservative management and medical and physical therapy, then rheumatologists recommend synovectomy. The efficiency of synovectomy in halting the ravages of the disease or in preventing recurrences has not been documented, but there is evidence that synovectomy delays, to a degree, damage to the cartilage. It may delay or prevent phase I from proceeding to phases II and III.[5,6]

Structural joint damage may be treated surgically by the insertion of a McIntosh prosthesis (Fig. 6–8). The aim of such a prosthesis is to alleviate pain, correct deformity, and increase range of motion. The hemiprosthesis also corrects excessive varus or valgus, depending on its specific placement in the joint. Restoring the width of the joint space results in a restoration of the proper alignment of the ligaments of the knee. Realignment of the joint allows the collateral ligaments to resume their normal physiological lengths.

Adequate quadriceps function is mandatory if the prosthesis is to be effective. However, insertion of a prosthesis allows the strength of the quadriceps muscle to be restored and maintained by therapeutic exercises since the muscles are no longer inhibited by pain and the limited range of motion of the joint.

Prosthesis must only be considered when synovectomy, debridement, and tibial osteotomy have been of no value and so little cartilage remains that bone rubs on bone. Prosthetic replacement is contraindicated when there has been previous plateau fracture, infection, or fusion; when there is concurrent neurotrophic arthritis; or when there is inability on the part of the patient to cooperate. Severe bone atrophy may also be a contraindication since the prosthesis may become unstable.

Total knee replacement is being performed more frequently with good results as the structural and surgical techniques improve. This is more thoroughly discussed in the section in this chapter devoted to degenerative knee joint disease.

As a last salvage procedure for an intractable, painful, unstable knee, an arthrodesis (fusion) can be considered. However, before surgery, the knee should be cast into a fully extended position to ascertain whether that relieves the pain, permits ambulation, and is psychologically acceptable to

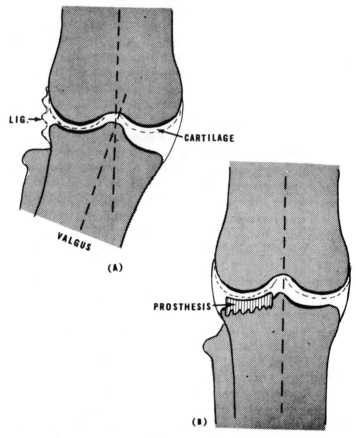

Figure 6–8. Treatment of degenerative arthritis with tibial plateau hemiprosthesis. (A) The usual valgus of the degenerated knee joint with marked narrowing of the lateral joint compartment. The capsule is redundant. (B) Insertion of the prosthesis straightens the knee and separates the lateral joint space.

the patient. Before fusing the involved knee, determine the competence of function of the patient's hands and arms, as well as the condition of the knee, hip, foot, and ankle of the contralateral leg. It must never be forgotten that a fusion is permanent and essentially irreversible.

OSTEOARTHRITIS OR OSTEOARTHROSIS (DEGENERATIVE ARTHRITIS)

Osteoarthritis, also commonly called degenerative arthritis and osteoarthrosis, is considered a sequela of traumatic and age-dependent degenerative changes which result in a loss of cartilage and impairment of function. Medicine remains frustrated in its attempt to specifically delineate the etiology of idiopathic osteoarthritis. Most recently, a genetic basis for degenerative arthritis has been offered, but this does not fully explain the condition other than to specify who among us may develop this degenerative condition.

Because of studies conducted during recent decades using biochemical, molecular biological, and ultrastructural techniques, the steps leading to degeneration are becoming more understandable, but the initial step in the etiology remains obscure. Radin and coworkers[7] postulate that this is because the mechanical and biological relationships have not been fully explored. Radin[8] deplores the fact that all research in the pathophysiology of degenerative joint disease has been slanted toward biochemistry and immunology *without* full acceptance and understanding of the mechanical aspect of joint pathology.

Osteoarthritis has been essentially classified as *primary* (idiopathic) or *secondary*, that is, a process related to infection, trauma, inflammation, metabolism, or aging. This meaningless classification further signifies the ambiguity of the process of degenerative osteoarthritis.

A joint, an articulation, provides movement between two bones with minimal effort. Joints provide support against gravity, but are also compressed because of the actions of the muscles that span and act on that joint.

It is well recognized that articular cartilage is very resistant to abrasion so long as some lubricant fluid remains within the joint.[9,10] The surface of articular cartilage is normally moist, consisting of about 80 percent water. The mechanical aspect of lubrication, which requires repeated compression and release for imbibition of nutrients, has been well documented. An adequate osmotic potential exists that allows the cartilage to "suck" fluid back when pressure is reduced. In addition, the size of the cartilage pores keeps the mucopolysaccharide molecules within the cartilage.

Synovial fluid is not an oil. It is a slow-flowing, viscous, thixotropic fluid composed of extremely large molecules. Because of its viscoelasticity, it is also an excellent shock absorber.

Hydrodynamic lubrication was initially described in 1888 in the engineering literature, but it remained for MacConaill[12] in 1932 to relate this concept to human synovial joints. His concept of "congruity versus incongruity" implies that relative movement of one part of a bearing surface of an asymmetrical joint[13] (Fig. 6–9) sucks lubricating fluid between the two adjacent bearing surfaces (Fig. 6–10).

Incongruity of the opposing joint surfaces and of the intra-articular structures such as the menisci augments the hydrodynamic lubricating mechanisms. Direct pressure on cartilage would not cause fluid to ooze out at the point of contact, but fluid does flow into incongruous joints and is spread by contact as the joint surfaces slide along. Articular cartilage is too

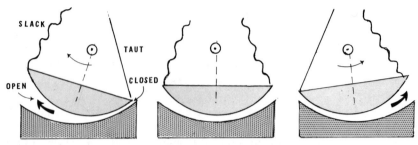

Figure 6–9. Asymmetrical joint surfaces. The asymmetrical joint surfaces of incongruous joints cause synovial fluid (*large arrow*) to flow toward the open articular area. The joint ligaments remain taut on the closing side and become slack on the opening side.

compliant under pressure and closes off the joint space, which violates the principle of joint lubrication within congruous joints.

The coefficient of friction in animal joints was found to be lower than that of machine bearings.[12] As long as the surfaces remained wet, the coefficient of lubrication remained low and allowed lubrication to proceed. Animal joints use what is called *boundary lubrication*, that is, layers of lubricating molecules stick to the opposing joint surfaces and glide on each

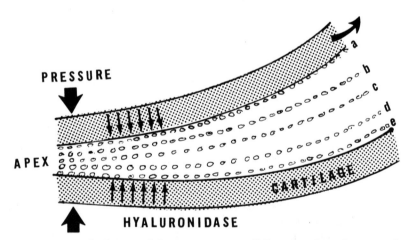

Figure 6–10. Hydrodynamic lubrication. Nonparallel wedge-shaped joint surfaces enclose lubricating fluid, some of which stays at the apex. The lubricating fluid moves in layers, first (a), then (b), (c), (d), and finally (e). The fluid moves at the same speed as the articulating bone but layers (a) and (e) adhere to both articular surfaces. A shear force between the layers causes deformation of the fluid.

The lubricant is both adhesive and viscous, being coated by hyaluronic acid created by the synovium and cartilage. Even without movement, layers remain between the two opposing joint surfaces.

other (see Fig. 6–10). Boundary lubrication occurs during low-weight-bearing conditions but not under heavy loads.

Hyaluronidase was considered to be the substance responsible for boundary lubrication. This is now in question. Recently a hyaluronidase-free glycoprotein has been discovered and thought to be the lubricant.[15]

McCutchen[16] established that joint lubrication was possible only if the enclosed fluid flowed ("weeped") from only one surface, causing extremely low friction. Since cartilage, along with its subchondral bone, contains 80 percent water, it weeps fluid and is an excellent lubricating mechanism.

Articular cartilage was initially considered to be inert tissue, maintaining only infusion and diffusion of fluids. It was believed that chondrocytes do not undergo mitotic division and hence could not repair cartilage (Fig. 6–11). Recent studies indicate that they do divide[17] and that cartilage can repair itself.[18]

Whether the surface of articular cartilage continues to be slowly worn away during life remains conjectural (Fig. 6–12). Wearing away is probably pathological and not merely an "aging process." However, articular cartilage is very susceptible to wear when subjected to oscillation and repeated

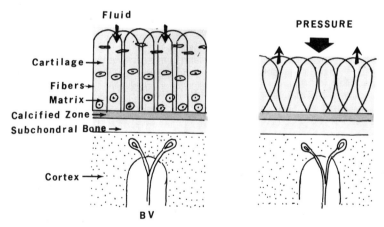

Figure 6–11. Cartilage nutrition. (*Left*) The "relaxed" cartilage has collagen fibers and chondrocyte cells within the matrix. These cells are active in the basal layers and flatten toward the periphery until they become flat and flake off when they exit the cartilage. The zone immediately below the cartilage is the calcified zone that does not permit the passage of blood vessels (BV) into the cartilage. Immediately under this zone is the subchondral bone and then the cortex. The blood vessels end as bulbs. In the relaxed state the cartilage is expanded and absorbs fluid (*small arrows*) from the synovial cavity.

(*Right*) The cartilage is compressed by gravity and muscular contraction (*large arrow*). This occurs because of compression of the collagen fiber "springs." Fluid is compressed from the cartilage to "weep" into the synovial cavity (*small arrows*).

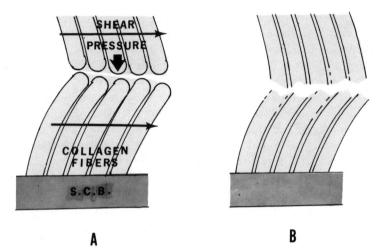

A   **B**

Figure 6–12. Shear deformation of cartilage. (A) The opposing cartilages of a moving joint cause the curving deformation of the collagen fibers. This shear force is augmented by compressive forces from gravity and muscular action. The underlying subchondral bone (S.C.B.) is shown. (B) The shear effect has caused a degeneration of the collagen fiber with irregularity of the cartilage matrix.

longitudinal loading. These mechanical factors lead to *fatigue* of the cartilage with resultant chemical alterations.

The surfaces of synovial joints that rub are made up of more than merely the cartilage. In fact is has been claimed that the friction resulting from cartilage rubbing on cartilage is "negligible."[19,20] The synovial tissues also play a vital role in joint lubrication and frictionless motion. Hyaluronidase is considered to essentially lubricate these periarticular soft tissues.[21] Hyaluronidase is also considered to add *adhesion* to the joint, keeping the articular surfaces together. Articular mechanics are complex but are gradually being described.

Articular cartilage tends to deform, causing resultant tension at its periphery. A constant clinical finding is the presence of cartilage degeneration in the load-bearing areas, implying that compression and shear play a vital role in degeneration. Cartilage, albeit resilient because of its viscoelastic properties, is too thin to be an effective shock absorber. Cartilage absorbs most of the shock at its bony union, which deforms on compression, and through the muscular ligamentous reaction to external stresses. It remains to be shown how the reaction time of the neuromuscular reaction to external stress influences degenerative injury of joint cartilage but it can be seen as a pertinent factor.

Although loads borne by joints come from weight bearing, most of the force on joints results from muscular contraction about the joint. In every activity of daily living, whether ambulation or sports activities, there is longitudinal stress applied along the axis of the skeleton. The muscles keep the body upright against gravity, which consumes most of our expended energy.[22] The muscles acting across the knee joint are alternately used for acceleration and deceleration, which places compressive stress and impact on the knee. The cartilage absorbs some portion of these forces, but the subchondral bone probably absorbs most of it.[23]

To summarize, degenerative joint changes are apparently the result of

1. Longitudinal forces, which include mechanical impact and muscular contraction
2. Cartilage compression
3. Impact on the subchondral bone, which results in microfractures[24] (Fig. 6–13)

The metabolism of the overlying cartilage thus becomes changed.[25] The pore size is altered, creating a change in the osmotic pressure and allowing the ground substance of the cartilage to flow out, but it does not adequately return on release of pressure. In addition, the matrix is changed chemically by the action of lysosomal lytic enzymes.

Experimental studies performed on animals, but undoubtedly applicable to humans, have revealed that superficial lacerations (not approaching the subchondral bone) do not progress or heal.[26] *Deep* lesions that violate the underlying bone plate undergo characteristic changes (Fig. 6–14).

Initially the defect fills with blood from the end plate blood vessels, which rapidly becomes organized into a fibrous clot. Some of the included blood cells change into fibroblasts within 10 days, and with chondrification,

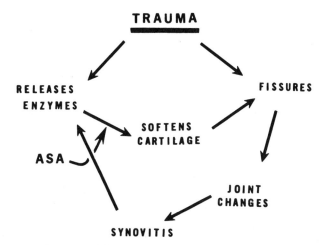

Figure 6–13. Schematic of the processes that help cause degenerative arthritis.

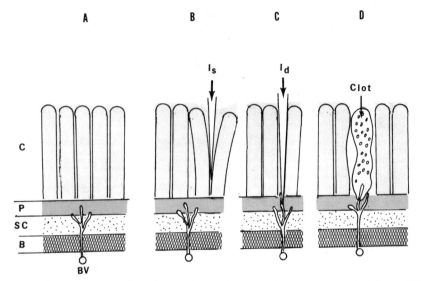

Figure 6–14. Response of cartilage to laceration to study the response to injury. (A) Normal cartilage (C) with a calcified plate (P), subchondral bone (SC), and bone cortex (B) that contains the blood vessels (BV).

(B) A shallow laceration (I_s) that does not reach the subchondral bone. Healing does not occur, nor is there progression of the damage.

(C) A deep laceration (I_D) that penetrates matrix and enters the subchondral bone plate. The blood vessels (BV) enter the area of laceration.

(D) Repair with the penetrated blood vessels forming a blood clot that contains cells and fibroblasts. This heals into a fibrocartilaginous tissue.

fibrocartilaginous tissue is formed. There is no evidence for tangential sliding of this newly formed fibrocartilage; it merely covers the defect and will remain there for years. The overlying cartilage demonstrates a dimple, with the remainder of the adjacent cartilage being normal in structure and function.

How these "traumata" occur remains the crux of the determination of cartilage pathology.[27] Normal joints are incongruous with areas of both contact and noncontact. These concepts of incongruity and lubrication have already been discussed. With increased loads (weight and muscular contraction), the contact areas become larger and become remodeled, gradually forming a more congruous joint. This joint now responds more to lesser loads. This gradual *molding* into a more congruous joint indicates why "aging" is involved in the evolution of osteoarthritic changes. Trauma can therefore be a shear force or direct laceration cleavage. The end result is a breakdown of the collagen fibers or a change in the cellular matrix, causing further irregularity of the gliding surfaces. The shear is aggravated by loss, failure, or deficiency of the ligaments and muscular components of the knee or damage to the menisci, all of which are discussed in the chapter related to each of these structures.

Chemical changes in the degenerated cartilage have been postulated. The concentration of proteoglycans is diminished and the collagen molecules do not change although their physical characteristics are altered.[28] They are larger in diameter except at the periphery, where they are frayed. There is an *increase* in their water content, the reason for which is, as yet, unknown.

There appears to be an increase in the levels of proteolytic enzymes, which have not been isolated or identified, but these enzymes have a role in cartilage degradation. The current understanding of the role of enzymes in degenerative osteoarthritis is summarized by Mankin.[26]

Treatment of the Osteoarthritic Knee

The pain of the osteoarthritic knee has been treated with oral nonsteroidal anti-inflammatory medication, which brings some relief to the patient. The use of aspirin must always be considered as an excellent anti-inflammatory medication when all the precautions have been exercised.

Repeated intra-articular injections of soluble steroids have resulted in some relief, but the results are extremely variable. Long-range benefit has not been ascertained. Inclusion of an anesthetic agent in the steroid solution has often led to excessive use of the knee, which is potentially detrimental.

Since osteoarthritis is postulated to result from repeated microtraumas that lead to thickening and resilience of the subchondral bone. Research projects using intra-articular administration (in rabbits) of antichondromucoprotein immune globulin has given some credence to this idea.[27,28] There is evidence that cells attempting to replenish the cartilage matrix are inhibited by the formation of adverse synovial enzymes created by cartilage breakdown, essentially an immunological breakdown.[29]

Soft tissue surgical procedures in animals have created lesions similar to those seen in human osteoarthritis, which bodes well for future solutions. These studies have also shown that cartilage *can* and *does* repair itself and that lytic enzymes are created, which may also lead to an antienzyme approach. Uridine diphosphate has been shown to enhance acceleration of proteoglycan synthesis (a cartilage reproduction enhancer).[30,31,32]

Injury to the thin membrane that covers the surface of articular cartilage, lamina splendens, may initiate damage to the cartilage. However, the damage is superficial and does not progress. An arthroscopic investigation can injure this membrane; therefore, this invasive procedure must be performed with care and gentleness. Because of this reaction from arthroscopy, the clinician should have a firm clinical reason for ordering or performing this procedure. Unless the exact diagnosis is not apparent and the expected treatment requires this diagnosis, merely to arthroscope "to see the inside of the joint" and confirm the clinical impression is unjustified. For arthroscopy to be justified, it must be ascertained that the contemplated diagnosis is not verifiable without arthroscopy and the condition found will conceivably benefit from "surgical intervention."

Excessive scraping of the cartilage during an arthroscopic procedure causes an elevation (heat) on bone scanning, which indicates inflammation, that is, a hypervascularity of the subchondral bone because the cartilage itself is avascular. Persistent pain has been reported after even a simple arthroscopic examination.

Treatment of the Acute and/or Early Degenerated Knee Joint

The alignment of the knee must be ascertained. If present, excessive varus or valgus must be addressed. A severely pronated foot or a foot in severe valgus may have a detrimental effect on the knee and should be corrected.[33]

Daily activities must be modified. Excessive athletic activities must be curtailed or eliminated until the acute phase has subsided. Resumption of these activities will depend on the exact sport, its potential damaging effects, and the psychological demands of the patient.

Modification of the environment must also be considered. For example, the heights of chairs, steps, and toilet seats that are used daily must be evaluated and corrected if necessary.

Muscle imbalance must be evaluated. Weakness of the knee extensors, with or without atrophy, must be ascertained and corrected by diligent daily resistive exercises. Weakness of the quadriceps muscle is undoubtedly the major muscular weakness of a symptomatic degenerated knee and must be determined. These issues have been discussed elsewhere in this book (Chap. 3). Exercises recommended for patellofemoral degenerative disease are described in Chapter 5.

Weakness of the hamstrings must also be ascertained and, if present, corrected. Hip abductor and adductor weakness occasionally exists, which should be corrected with appropriate strengthening exercises.

Immobilization of an acutely inflamed knee is frequently advocated. Brief immobilization is undoubtedly valuable. How "brief" is uncertain, but it must be remembered that within 3 weeks of immobilization, atrophy of the quadriceps can already be measured. Rest for a few days is acceptable, then non-weight-bearing isometric exercises are indicated (see Chap. 3).

An elastic prosthetic support may permit weight bearing in early stages while more definitive measures are evaluated. Use of a cane or even crutches is indicated when the condition is acute and severe.

Local use of ice is recommended for edema of the inflamed knee because this modality results in (1) hypalgesia, (2) diminution of hyperemia,

(3) decrease of histamine nociceptors, and (4) decrease of sympathetic nervous system irritation (Fig. 6–15). Ice cubes or chips enclosed in a plastic bag can be wrapped around the knee for periods of 20 minutes several times a day. However, after 48 hours moist heat should be used instead of ice. Local moist heat brings new blood, and therefore nutrition, via the synovium to the cartilage.

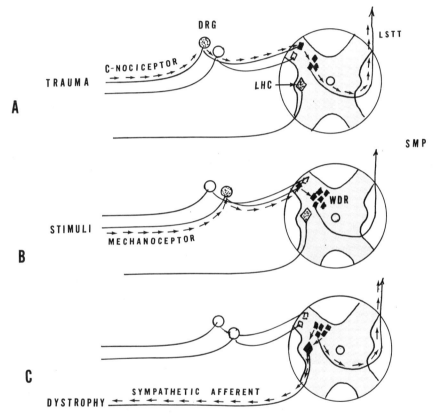

Figure 6–15. (A) Peripheral trauma initiates afferent nociceptor impulses that enter the dorsal columns in the substantia gelatinosum through the dorsal root ganglia (DRG) and transfer to the contralateral lateral spinal thalamic tracts (LSTT) then ascend to the thalamus. LHC is the site of the lateral horn cells from which eminate the efferant sympathetic impulses.

(B) The mechanoceptor impulses that are transmitted via Ia and myelinated fibers enter the area of the cord containing wide dynamic range (WDR) neurons which have become hyperirritable from the nociceptor bombardment as in (A). This constitutes sympathetic maintained pain (SMP).

(C) Via a mononeural arc the afferent impulses now stimulate the lateral horn cells (LHC) and transmit efferent sympathetic impulses to cause peripheral vasomotor changes known as dystrophy.

Alternate compression-relaxation of the knee cartilage is needed to maintain nutrition and regeneration of damaged cartilage. Walking is to be encouraged but must be modified depending on the severity and stage of degeneration. Arthritis of the knee decreases the velocity of walking, rate of knee flexion and extension, and range of motion.[34]

Contracture of the knee joint is a frequent event in degenerative arthritis of the knee. The knee may experience slight flexion and contraction, preventing full extension, or there may be persistent extension. Both have an adverse effect on gait. Analysis of the knee in gait is fully discussed in Chapter 9. Only pertinent factors will be alluded to here.

When examining a knee with early degenerative arthritis, the full range of motion, as compared to the other, "normal" knee, must be determined. Active and passive exercises can correct early capsular contraction or muscle fascial contracture.

Continuous passive motion (CPM) has been advocated for postoperative patients with articular cartilage injuries.[35] CPM is also desirable for the nonoperated knee. It is desirable that the patient obtain a home CPM unit, but if one is not available, then daily flexion-extension, non-weight-bearing exercises can be instituted. A bicycle fulfills CPM-type of exercises.

If the knee if slightly flexed and fails to fully extend, the gait is described as a "short leg" limp. If the contracture is less than 30°, the limp is noted only at a high walking speed. If flexion contracture is greater than 30°, the limp will be noted at lower speeds. A knee contracted in full extension does not flex at the midstance phase. Thus the gait appears similar to the one seen in an individual whose legs are of unequal length.

A knee that bears full weight with a slight degree of flexion is physiologically impaired and places stress on the weight-bearing joint and impairs the gait. Bracing may be needed to correct a severe contracture (Fig. 6–16). This brace may be applied only at night, all day, or a combination of both. Its use must always be accompanied by active-passive exercises to prevent further contracture and atrophy.

Treatment of Severe and Chronic Degenerative Arthritis

Surgical intervention via the arthroscope is now accepted in the treatment of acute or chronic full-thickness defects in cartilage. After evaluation and debridement, minor fractures at the base of the defects are surgically induced. This is intended to enhance the resultant blood clot that normally occurs but surgically is considered as "controlled" in degree and depth. Impact loading is minimized postoperatively by the use of crutches and the affected knee is placed on a CPM program for 8 weeks.[35]

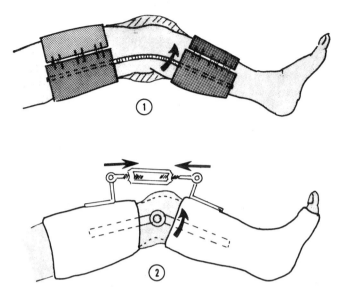

Figure 6–16. Corrective splinting of hemophilic arthritis. (*1*) During the acute phase of hemarthrosis, a splint, consisting of a thigh and a lower leg thermoplastic shell held by Velcro straps, can be connected with a flexible wire that can be bent to gradually extend the knee. The knee is visible and change can be made immediately if there is any increase in hemorrhaging. (*2*) A plaster cast, hinged at the knee, can be made for chronic fibrous contracture of the knee in varying degrees of flexion. Gradual extension is obtained by a dorsal turnbuckle that can be turned gradually several times a day or a few degrees every other day as tolerated.

The affected knee should not bear any weight. This must be stressed because any weight bearing causes a loss of the clot or causes the clot to become a hypervascular type of fibrous tissue. If there is no weight bearing for 8 weeks, the clot becomes a spindle-cell avascular tissue. This "repaired" cartilage resembles normal cartilage, but the long-term effect of this procedure has not been, as yet, documented. CPM and the lack of weight bearing appear essential for a successful outcome. Tibial osteotomy is advocated by some to realign the lower extremity and thus rebalance the stresses caused by gravity on the knee.

Total knee replacement has clinical results that equal or exceed the results of total hip replacement in terms of pain relief, improved function, and 10-year survival.[36] The most successful designs for replacement of both surfaces of the knee joint follow the hinge designs of Walldius[37] (Fig. 6–17). It is now a valid replacement for an arthrodesis (fusion) of the knee, which eliminates the pain but is a difficult decision, both cosmetically and functionally, for the patient.

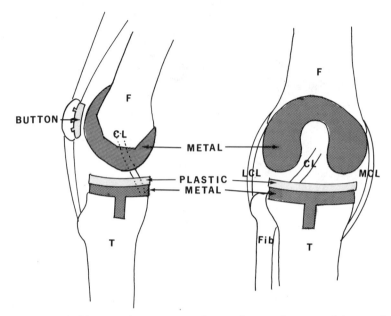

Figure 6–17. Total knee replacement prosthesis. The metal aspects of the prosthesis cover the distal portion of the femur (F) and the end of the tibia (T). There is a polyethylene plastic-bearing surface (plastic) between the metalic aspects of the two surfaces. The patella is replaced by a polyethylene button.

The medial collateral ligament (MCL), lateral collateral ligament (LCL), and cruciate ligaments (CL) are retained. Fib = fibula.

The indications for total knee arthroplasty are excruciating pain and failure to respond to conservative treatment. The patient's age, weight, desired level of activities, and complicating medical problems must be considered.

The contraindications for total knee replacement are:

Youth. Tibial osteotomy may be preferable.

Obesity. Excessive weight shortens the life of the total knee implant.

Painful patellofemoral degenerative arthritis. Patellectomy may present a more desirable intervention.

Pre-existing bony fusion of the knee. This is a relative contraindication since the expected range of motion after the arthroplasty is usually limited. Especially since a fused knee is usually free of pain, the advisability of a total replacement is questionable.

Pyogenic infection. This constitutes a significant contraindication.

Extensive athletic activities. The patient's desire to partake in athletic activity may not be satisfied after a total knee replacement, and this must be taken into account before a decision is made.

HEMOPHILIC ARTHRITIS

Hemophilia is an inherited hemorrhagic condition that is maternally transmitted to male offspring. Essentially, the disease is a failure of the blood to clot. Hemarthrosis, bleeding into joints, is seen in 80 to 90 percent of patients with hemophilia and presents a major symptom of this bleeding disorder.

The onset of hemophilia is usually between the ages of 4 to 10, when there is excessive and uncontrollable bleeding as a sequela of trauma. In this age group, the knee is a frequent site of trauma, so knee hemarthrosis is often the first indication of this disease. If there is repeated, prolonged, and excessive bleeding, there are tests that can confirm the presence of this disease.

The acute hemarthrotic knee becomes painful, swollen, warm, and markedly tender. Discoloration may be noted, indicating bleeding. There may be a related fever and leukocytosis. If the bleeding is mild, the joint may return to normal within a few days with no sequelae or residual. In severe hemarthrosis the knee may remain inflamed for weeks or months.

Repeated hemarthrosis leads to hemosiderosis (a deposit of hemosiderin, granules consisting of ill-defined complexes of ferric hydroxides, polysaccharides, and proteins) of the synovium, gradual degeneration of the cartilage, and thickening of the capsule and other periarticular soft tissues. The sequelae of joint damage appear to be (1) cartilage damage resulting from excessive, unremitting pressure from the increased bloody synovial fluid, (2) impairment of the nutritive aspect of the synovial fluid, and (3) possible toxic elements within the hemophilic blood, which have not yet been confirmed.

Repetitive and persistent hemarthrosis thins the cartilage. Subchondral cysts occur, forming a pannus that contains fibroblasts. Ultimately a fibrous ankylosis may form (Fig. 6–18).

Contracture may result from this fibrous tissue invasion and from the thickening of the capsule. Flexion contracture predominates, but gradually knee motion may be limited in all directions and may even be ankylosed in extension.

X-ray studies done in the early stages of the disease reveal that the bony edges may become irregular and the epiphysis may hypertrophy.[38] Many joints may remain normal in spite of numerous bouts of hemarthrosis, but 50 percent are considered to undergo permanent articular changes. Bleeding may progress into the periarticular muscular tissues, causing a blood tumor or a *hemophilic pseudocyst*.[39] Bleeding into muscle tissue may cause destructive changes of the muscle. Bleeding may also progress into the periosteum and into the bone of the thigh or tibia.

The prevention of any trauma is mandatory, albeit difficult, in young active males. Guidance and psychological therapy assist in this venture.

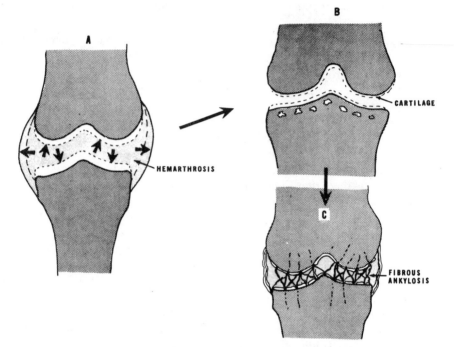

Figure 6–18. Hemophilic arthritis. (A) Hemarthrosis with bloody effusion distending the capsule and putting pressure (*arrows*) against the cartilage of the femur and the tibia. (B) If there is persistence or frequent recurrence of hemarthrosis, the cartilage thins. (C) Chronic stage with fibrous reaction within the bloody effusion, organization of the hemorrhagic effusion, fibrous invasion through the damaged cartilage, and ultimately fibrous ankylosis.

Treatment[38] of the hemophiliac requires immediate plasma infusion, vitamin K, and all other current therapies.

Active local treatment of the knee cannot begin until the bleeding is under control. During this phase, a posterior mold splint should be used to rest the joint and to allow ambulation. Local ice packs applied frequently during the day may relieve pain and diminish further bleeding. A firm yet gentle compression dressing applied before significant swelling occurs is of value.

Aspiration of the joint is beneficial; however, there must be medical control of the bleeding first since invasion may cause more bleeding or a recurrence of bleeding. Intra-articular injection of steroids or hyaluronidase has been claimed to thin the synovial fluid[40] and minimize proliferative changes of the synovium and further progression of fibrosis. How the steroids or hyaluronidase accomplish this feat remains conjectural.

Injection of hyaluronidase must be performed aseptically. A measured amount of joint fluid is aspirated, and an equal amount of hyaluronidase with a 1 percent procaine (or a derivative) solution is added and reinjected into the joint. Only as much fluid as is needed to form the hyaluronidase solution should be aspirated. Following the intra-articular injection, a firm elastic bandage is evenly applied and the joint rested in an elevated position for several hours. Persistence of pain is an indication for a repeated infusion in 24 hours.

Once the pain has stopped or is significantly diminished, gentle, passive range of motion exercises and gradual *isometric* quadriceps contraction can begin. Gradually isotonic contractions are added to slowly achieve the full range of motion, *especially extension*. Early ambulation usually requires a splint support for the first 24 to 48 hours.

Chronic adhesive capsulitis is feared because ultimate surgical correction in a patient with a bleeding tendency causes apprehension. Prevention and nonsurgical correction are desirable. During the acute phases of hemorrhaging, a padded splint with both halves held by a flexible wire (see Fig. 6–16) will assist in maintaining extension and permit some degree of active flexion. If the contracture appears inflexible, the inclusion of hinges permits slow, gradual extension of the knee. During splinting the knee must undergo active isometric and guarded isotonic exercises by the patient. Hydrotherapy is valuable if available. Exercises in a warm pool are usually well tolerated and are effective.

GOUTY ARTHRITIS

Gout is a hereditary metabolic disease that is maternally transmitted and that predominantly affects males. Clinically the disease becomes apparent in adult life between the ages of 35 to 50. Many relatives of patients with gout have hyperuricemia but never develop clinical manifestations.

Uric acid is known to be a threshold substance formed by the body, eliminated by the renal glomeruli, circulated in the blood, and reabsorbed by the kidney tubules. An impaired rate of absorption and elimination leads to clinical gout.

There are five postulated internal dysfunctions that lead to an increase of uric acid in tissue fluids:

1. Diminished excretion by the kidneys
2. Decreased glomerular filtration
3. Increased reabsorption by the renal tubules
4. Excessive formation of urates as a result of faulty metabolism
5. Diminished destruction of urates by faulty enzymes

An excess of urates in the blood does not constitute gout until the urates are deposited in mesenchymal tissues. What creates these abnormalities remains obscure. Urate crystals are prone to become deposited in avascular tissues rather than vascular tissues, which is why there is a predilection for urate deposit in cartilage, bursae, ligaments, tendons, and the epiphyseal portion of bone. Tophi (local accumulations of urates) are conspicuously absent from muscle, lungs, liver, nervous tissues, and (surprisingly) kidneys. Tophi are absent in less than 50 percent of patients with gouty arthritis, yet in joints the urate crystals are deposited in the superficial layers of the cartilage with resultant cartilage fibrillation. The cartilage overlying the urate deposit becomes destroyed (Fig. 6–19), while the crystals are released into the joint and the synovial fluid.

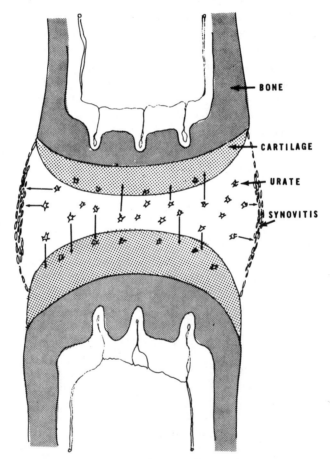

Figure 6–19. Schematic explanation of gouty arthritis. The exact mechanism of gouty arthritis is not verified. The currently accepted theory is that urate crystals form in the synovial fluid and penetrate the outer layer of the cartilage, depositing crystals there. Urate crystals also irritate the synovial layer, causing synovitis. The hypothesis that urates migrate via the subchondral epiphyseal bone is not currently accepted.

While still within the superficial layers of the cartilage, the urate accumulations (intracartilaginous tophi) become surrounded by granular tissue containing leukocytes, round cells, and giant cells. These tophi are surrounded by edematous and hyperemic tissue, and they gradually soften as the crystals are released into the synovium.

During an acute attack of gouty arthritis, the joint becomes swollen, reddened, and tense, with the overlying skin becoming taut and shiny. Onset is usually sudden, with severe pain, and rapid swelling and discoloration. Characteristically, gouty arthritis occurs in "one" joint, which is of diagnostic significance in differentiating it from an acute attack of rheumatoid arthritis. Also of differential diagnostic significance is that in RA there is often symmetrical and bilateral multiarticular involvement, predominantly in women who are also usually emaciated, "sick" patients. In gouty arthritis, symptoms not only occur in adult males and are uniarticular, but serum uric acid is elevated and crystals can be found in aspirated joint fluid.

Attacks are believed to result from trauma, overexertion, dietary or alcoholic excesses, surgical procedures elsewhere in the body, or severe diuresis from excessive use of diuretics. However, many acute exacerbations have no discernible cause.

X-ray studies of gouty arthritic joints are not pathognomonic. They reveal similar changes to those noted in studies of rheumatoid and degenerative arthritis. When subchondral cysts are noted on x-ray films, they are probably masses (tophi) of urate crystals.

Treatment is prophylactic with regard to systemic hyperuricemia.[39] The following are common recommendations:

Avoidance of purine-rich foods and fats
Decrease in body weight
Avoidance of diuretics and salicylates, which encourage the retention of uric acid, during the acute stage

Probenecid in doses of 0.5 g, three times daily, is the most commonly prescribed uricosuric medication. Renal disease is a contraindication for many uricosuric medications. Allopurinol in doses of 300 mg, once daily, is effective when the uric acid blood level is above 10 mg/100 ml. It must be remembered that patients with hyperuricemia may never develop gout and that patients with essentially normal blood uric acid levels may do so. During an acute attack, *nonsteroidal anti-inflammatory drugs* (NSAIDs) afford relief.

The involved knee should be treated symptomatically; it responds well to medication without the need for local physiatric therapy. If the pain is severe and disabling, the knee should be immobilized with a posterior molded splint and bed rest is advisable. Cold compresses are effective. If there is marked effusion, aspiration will diminish the symptoms and hasten recovery. Compression dressings are usually poorly tolerated. Recovery from an acute exacerbation usually occurs with no residual. Repeated bouts of gouty arthritis may ultimately cause degenerative changes similar to those of idiopathic degenerative arthritis described earlier in this chapter.

PSEUDOGOUT (CHONDROCALCINOSIS)

Pseudogout is a disorder where calcium-containing salts are deposited in articular cartilages of one or more joints. These salts include calcium pyrophosphate, calcium hydroxyapatite, and calcium orthophosphate. Pseudogout is essentially a crystal-induced arthritis (chondrocalcinosis) and occurs mostly in the elderly who may already have significant osteoarthritis.

This metabolic abnormality may be associated with hyperparathyroid disease, alkaptonuria, hemachromatosis, hepatolenticular degeneration (Wilson's disease), or acromegaly, or it may essentially be an idiopathic familial metabolic disorder. Many elderly diabetics exhibit calcinosis.

Clinically, pseudogout may be a smoldering arthritis that resembles osteoarthritis. There is intense inflammation of one or more joints during an acute attack. Onset is abrupt and usually lasts 2 weeks. Chronic arthritis has been known to occur.

The diagnosis is made by observing characteristic crystals (calcium pyrophosphate) in the aspirated synovial fluid.[40] They are rod-shaped crystals that are best observed under polarized light although they can be seen under an ordinary light microscope. In chronic effusions, the crystals are both intracellular and extracellular. The condition is best recognized radiologically[43]; calcifications can be seen within the cartilages, tendons, and bursae.

Treatment consists of combating the inflammation caused by the uricemia for which it appears to be specific. Aspiration of fluid from the inflamed joint often gives the patient immediate relief. Intra-articular injection of steroids may also be helpful. Rehabilitation treatment is merely supportive and symptomatic.

PYOGENIC ARTHRITIS

Suppurative arthritis is usually secondary to septicemia or to local invasion of a cellular infection. Clinically there is an acute onset with a hot, painful, swollen, red joint and systemic evidence of infection, including fever and leukocytosis.

Aspiration of the joint fluid reveals a thick, opaque, turbid fluid that reveals, on microscopic examination, cellular components consistent with infection. Culture of the fluid reveals the specific organism responsible.

The precise antibiotic is then administered both orally, intramuscularly, or intra-articularly, depending on the identity of the causative organism. Treatment involves rest of the joint, including posterior splinting, and hot, moist compresses are valuable. As soon as inflammation begins to subside, gentle, passive range of motion and isometric quadriceps exercises must be instituted.

BURSITIS

There are numerous bursae about the knee (Fig. 6–20). These bursae may become inflamed as a result of trauma or from repeated activities. They may be acute, recurrent, or chronic. When acute, they present a local swelling with palpable fluidity, local tenderness, and redness. They are clinically discernible as bursae and not as intra-articular swelling.

The prepatellar bursa lies between the skin and the outer surface of the patella. It frequently results from the direct trauma of a fall on the bent knee or merely from kneeling. The patella is seen and directly palpable, being swollen, tender, and inflamed. Pain can be intensified by direct pressure or tension on the skin, especially with full knee flexion.

Treatment of this prepatellar bursa is usually conservative—local heat and restricted activities. Aspiration may be needed if the swelling persists, but rarely is it necessary to incise and drain the cyst. A pressure dressing after aspiration ensures adhesion of the inflamed walls of the bursa and helps prevent any recurrence.

Deep infrapatellar bursitis usually occurs from overactivity, such as doing many deep knee bends and squats. Direct trauma is infrequent since the bursa is well protected by the overlying infrapatellar tendon and the underlying fat pad. Diagnostically, tenderness is elicted by pressure *behind* the patella or by forceful knee flexion or active quadriceps extension. Treatment also involves rest, immobilization, restricted activities, and local heat. Oral NSAIDs are of value. Aspiration with or without intrabursal steroid injection is indicated if the pain and tenderness persist. Excision is rarely needed but should be considered if the bursitis remains and disability persists.

Posterior bursitis is a cystic tumor in the popliteal space. This tumor is termed a popliteal, posterior bursitis, a synovial cyst, a Baker's cyst, a semimembranous or gastrocnemius membranous bursitis; 7 to 50 percent of these cysts communicate with the knee joint capsule. Arthrography has revealed this "communication" which implies that these cysts are synovial herniations that result from trauma and intra-articular effusions from various sources.

Treatment of these posterior bursae requires determination of the precise cause of the effusion of the capsule and the bursa. The original

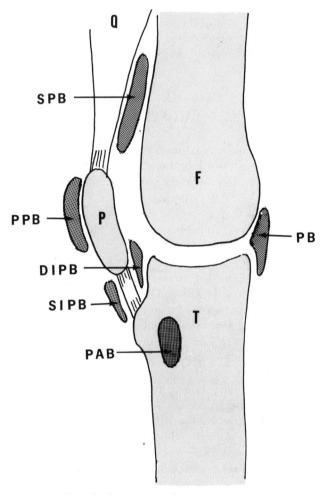

Figure 6–20. Bursae about the knee joint. The figure depicts the region of the bursa about the knee.

    F = Femur
    Q = Quadriceps and its tendons
    T = Tibia
  SPB = Suprapatellar bursa
  PPS = Prepatellar bursa
DIPB = Deep infrapatellar bursa
 SIPB = Superficial infrapatellar bursa
 PAB = Pes anserinus bursa
   PB = Popliteal bursa (a herniation of the capsule)

excision and/or aspiration of the cyst is no longer tenable but if the cyst is persistent and disabling, it may be surgically excised.[44,45]

REFERENCES

1. Swezey, RL: Rehabilitation in arthritis and allied conditions. In Kotte, FJ and Lehman, JF (eds): Krusen's Handbook of Physical Medicine and Rehabilitation, ed 4. WB Saunders, Philadelphia, 1990, p 679.
2. Mills, K: Pathology of the knee joint in rheumatoid arthritis. J Bone Joint Surg 52B:746, 1970.
3. Rodnan, GP, McEwen, C, and Wallace, S: Rheumatoid Arthritis: Primer on the Rheumatic Diseases, ed 7. Arthritis Foundation, Atlanta, 1973, section 7, p 25.
4. Cailliet, R: Foot and Ankle Pain, ed 2. FA Davis, Philadelphia, 1977.
5. Goldie, IF: Synovectomy in rheumatoid arthritis: A general review and an eight year follow-up of synovectomy in fifty rheumatoid patients. Semin Arthritis Rheum 3:219, 1974.
6. Arthritis Foundation Committee on Evaluation of Synovectomy: Multicenter evaluation of synovectomy in the treatment of rheumatoid arthritis. Arthritis Rheum 20:765–771, 1977.
7. Radin, EL, Igor, L, and Rose, RM: Mechanical factors in the aetiology of osteoarthrosis. Ann Rheum Dis (Suppl) 34:132, 1975.
8. Radin, EL: The physiology and degeneration of joints. Semin Arthritis Rheum 2:245, 1972–1973.
9. Radin, EL and Paul, IL: Arthritis Rheum 13:139, 1970.
10. Swann, DA, et al: Role of hyaluronic acid in joint lubrication. Ann Rheum Dis 33:318, 1974.
11. Cailliet, R: Mechanics of Joints, Arthritis and Physical Medicine, Vol 11. Waverly Press, Baltimore, 1969, p 17.
12. MacConaill, MA: The functions of intra-articular fibrocartilages, with special reference to the knee and inferior radio-ulnar joints. J Anat 66:210, 1932.
13. Cailliet, R: Shoulder Pain, ed 3. FA Davis, Philadelphia, 1991, p 1.
14. Jones, ES: Joint lubrication. Lancet 1:1426, 1934.
15. Radin, EL, Swann, DA, and Weisser, PA: Separation of a hyaluronate-free lubricating fraction from synovial fluid. Nature (London) 228:377, 1970.
16. McCutchen, CW: Mechanism of animal joints. Sponge hydrodynamic and weeping bearings. Nature 84:1284, 1959.
17. Mankin, HJ: Mitosis in articular cartilage of immature rabbits: A histologic, stathmokinetic (colchicinic) and autoradiographic study. Clin Orthop 34:170, 1964.
18. Kettunen, KO: Skin arthroplasty: In light of animal experiments with special reference to functional metaplasia of connective tissue. Acta Orthop Scand 29:9, 1958.
19. Smith, JW: Observations on the postural mechanism of the human knee joint. J Anat 90:236, 1956.
20. Johns, RJ and Wright, V: Relative importance of various tissues in joint stiffness. J Appl Physiol 17:824, 1962.
21. Radin, EI, Swann, DA, and Schottsteadt, ES: The lubrication of synovial membrane. Ann Rheum Dis 30:322, 1971.
22. Elftman, H: Biomechanics of muscle with particular attention to studies of gait. J Bone Joint Surg 48A:363, 1966.
23. Radin, IL and Tolkoff, MJ: Subchondral bone changes in patients with early degenerative arthritis. Arth Rheum 13:400, 1970.
24. Radin, EL: Trabecular microfractures in response to stress: The possible mechanism of Wolff's Law. Orthopaedic Surgery and Traumatology: Proceedings of the 12th Congress of the International Society of Orthopaedic Surgery and Traumatology, Tel Aviv. Exerpta Medica, Amsterdam, October 9–12, 1972, p 59.

25. Coutts, RD: Symposium: The diagnosis and treatment of injuries involving the articular cartilage. Contemp Ortho 19:401, 1989.

26. Mankin, HJ: The reaction of articular cartilage to injury and osteoarthritis, medical progress. New Engl J Med 291:12, 1974 and 291:1335, 1974.

27. Bullough, P, Goodfellow, J, and O'Connor, J: The relationship between degenerative changes and load bearing in the human hip. J Bone Joint Surg 55A:746, 1973.

28. Weiss, C: Ultrastructure characteristics of osteoarthritis. Fed Proc 32:1459, 1973.

29. Eguro, H and Goldner, L: Antigenic properties of chondromucoprotein and inducibility of experimental arthritis by antichondromucoprotein immune globulin. J Bone Joint Surg (in press).

30. Fell, HB and Jubb, RW: The effect of synovial tissue on the breakdown of articular cartilage in organ culture. Arth Rheum 20:1359, 1977.

31. Ehrlich, MG, et al: Uridine diphosphate (UDP) stimulation of protein-polysaccharide production: A preliminary report. J Bone Joint Surg 56A:1239, 1974.

32. Thompson, RC and Robinson, HJ: Articular cartilage matrix metabolism (current concepts review). J Bone Joint Surg 63A:327, 1981.

33. Cailliet, R: Foot and Ankle Pain. FA Davis, Philadelphia, 1983, p 89.

34. Brinkmann, JR and Perry, J: Rate and range of knee motion during ambulation in healthy and arthritic subjects. Phys Ther 65:1055, 1985.

35. Salter, RB, et al: The biologic effects of continuous passive motion on healing of full thickness defects in articular cartilage: An experimental study in the rabbit. J Bone Joint Surg 62A:1232, 1980.

36. Harris, WH and Sledge, CB: Total hip and knee replacement, medical progress. New Eng J Med 323:801, 1990.

37. Walldius, B: Arthroplasty of the knee joint using endoprosthesis. Acta Orthop Scand (Suppl) 24:17, 1957.

38. Ghormley, RK and Clegg, RS: Bone and joint changes in hemophilia. J Bone Joint Surg 30A:589, 1948.

39. Steel, WM, Duthie, RB, and O'Connor, BT: Hemophilic cysts: Report of five cases. J Bone Joint Surg 51B:614, 1969.

40. Smith, CF, et al: Long-term management and rehabilitation in hemophilia. Project report. PH Grant 110-91. Orthopedic Hospital, Los Angeles, 1969.

41. Kendall, PH: Arthritis and Physical Medicine. Waverly Press, Baltimore, 1969, p 205.

42. McCarty, DJ, Kohn, NN, and Faires, JS: The significance of calcium phosphate crystal in the synovial fluid of arthritic patients: The pseudogout syndrome. I. Clinical aspect. Ann Intern Med 56:711, 1962.

43. Martel, W, et al: A roentgenologically distinctive arthropathy in some patients with the pseudogout syndrome. Amer J Roentgenol Radium Ther Nucl Med 109:587, 1970.

44. Wilson, PD, Eyre-Brook, AL, and Francis, JD: A clinical and anatomical study of the semimembranosus bursa in relation to popliteal cyst. J Bone Joint Surg 20:963, 1938.

45. Wolfe, RD and Colloff, B: Popliteal cysts, an arthrographic study and review of the literature. J Bone Joint Surg 54A:1057, 1972.

CHAPTER 7

Fractures About the Knee Joint

No treatise of the knee would be complete without a discussion of fractures about the knee joint. Some of these fractures may be very complicated and present difficulties in their management; thus full dissertation of all these aspects cannot be covered in this brief chapter. Only basic types and basic principles of their management will be discussed.

Fractures about the knee may be classified in various categories: fractures of the distal end of the femur, proximal end of the tibia, and the patella. Fractures of the distal end of the femur may be divided into supracondylar, intercondylar, and condylar (Fig. 7–1). Fractures of the tibial plateau may be divided into those (1) involving the lateral condyle or the medial condyle, (2) with or without comminution or displacement, and (3) with variable degrees of depression.

Fractures about the knee must also be evaluated with respect to the injury sustained by the cartilage: chondral fractures involving only the articular cartilage or osteochondral fractures involving the articular cartilage and the underlying subchondral bone. Sudden violent stress can cause avulsion fracture in which a fragment of bone is avulsed by its attachment to a tendon or ligament.

Fractures can be caused by torsion injuries that were incurred when the fixed foot was internally or externally rotated in relationship to the femur, by direct violence, or by cartilage damage secondary to subluxation of the patella.

Symptoms consist of effusion (hemarthrosis), pain, localized tenderness, crepitation, locking, and varying degrees of disability. X-ray films may be diagnostic but may be unrewarding in chondral fractures. Arthrography may show a radiolucent filling defect when a fracture is suspected. Management obviously depends on the exact mechanism of fracture, the alignment of the fragments, the articular integrity, and proper joint surface alignment. Basic

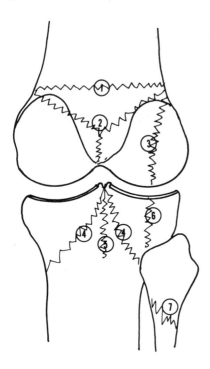

Figure 7-1. Fractures about the knee joint: fractures of distal femur and proximal tibia. *1*, Supracondylar fracture; *2*, intercondylar fracture Y type; *3*, condylar fracture of femur; *4*, condylar fracture of tibial plateau; *5*, intercondylar vertical fracture of tibial plateau; *6*, condylar fracture of medial or lateral tibia; and *7*, fibular fracture.

principles must underlie all treatment such as removal of fragment, removal of an associated meniscus tear, replacement of the fragment with internal fixation, and reconstruction of the extensor mechanism.

FRACTURES OF DISTAL END OF FEMUR

Anatomically, the distal end of the femur comprises two large rounded condyles covered with cartilage (see Chap. 1). Muscular attachment about the joint influences the resultant fracture fragments and their alignment. The gastrocnemius muscle pulls the distal fragment posteriorly (Fig. 7–2) toward the nerves and the blood vessels of the popliteal fossa. The collateral ligaments are frequently involved in the mechanism of fracture and must always be fully evaluated in determination of the extent of the fracture. Effusion (hemarthrosis) of the knee joint usually is present. Soft tissue must always be considered in prolonged immobilization with fragments in proper alignment because of the possibility of muscular atrophy (quadriceps femorus) and intra-articular adhesions. Improper realignment of the cartilage surface may lead to ultimate arthritic changes (a complication possible even with the best alignment).

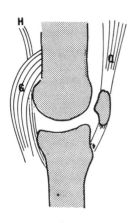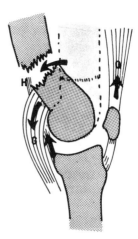

Figure 7–2. Muscular action upon fracture fragments: supracondylar fracture. (*Left*) Muscular action about the knee joint. (*Right*) Action of the gastrocnemius, pulling the distal fragment posteriorly into the popliteal fossa, and the hamstring and quadriceps pulling longitudinally to shorten the femur.
G = Gastrocnemius
H = Hamstrings
Q = Quadriceps

Supracondylar Fractures

This type of fracture is usually caused by direct violence or torsion stress. Usually there is displacement of the fragments (see Fig. 7–2) caused by muscular action, the gastrocnemius pulling the distal fragment posteriorly into the fossa and the hamstrings and quadriceps shortening the length of the femur.

Management may be closed reduction or open reduction, with the former usually possible and desirable.[1] Alignment is attempted on a fracture table and with skeletal traction. If the joint is distended with blood, it is aspirated under sterile technique. The hip is flexed (45° to 60°) (Fig. 7–3). The flexed lower leg tends to reduce the posterior displacement and manual pressure completes this displacement. After reduction, a plaster spica is applied with the knee in the flexed position and the wires incorporated into the plaster. Wires are usually removed in 4 to 6 weeks and the cast removed in 6 to 8 weeks.

In cases that defy reduction, continuous traction in a Bohler-Braun splint may be necessary. The principles are the same as those just discussed. The gained position of reduction can usually be maintained with 10 to 12 lb of traction, but as much as 20 to 25 lb of traction for 24 to 48 hours may be

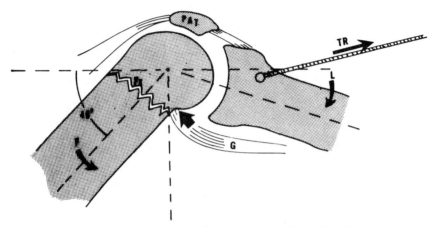

Figure 7–3. Management of supracondylar fracture. This hip is flexed 45°. The lower leg, by its weight, reduces the lower femoral fragment assisted by manual pressure (*thick arrow*) upward against the distal fragment. Traction (TR) is initially applied to separate the fragments. A spica cast is applied with hip and knee flexed, and the pin is incorporated.

necessary. Because muscular atrophy of the quadriceps occurs early, exercises of the isometric type (quad setting) should be started immediately and immobilization in plaster should not be kept any longer than absolutely necessary.

After removal of the spica plaster, the leg may be placed in balanced suspension and more active exercises begun. Within 2 to 4 weeks, the quadriceps should be reasonably strong and the fracture adequately healed to permit weight bearing in a walking caliper splint. Obviously, time factors are determined by age and severity of fracture as well as patient cooperation.

When closed reduction is not possible, open reduction may be necessary.

Intercondylar Fractures

These fractures of the femur (Fig. 7–4) may be of the Y or T type; they are more severe than supracondylar fractures. Soft tissue injury may be extensive. The fracture may be exceedingly unstable with reduction and maintenance of the reduction difficult.

Management (Fig. 7–5) is basically that of traction to regain the length of the femur after aspiration of the joint hemorrhage, manual or clamp manipulation to approximate the condylar fragments, plaster in the reduced position, and *immediate periodic supervised quadriceps exercises.* Postreduction care is similar to that of supracondylar fracture. Surgical (open)

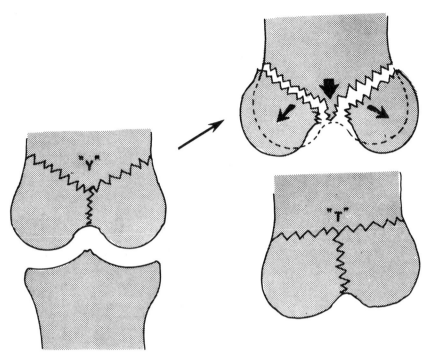

Figure 7–4. Intercondylar fractures of the distal femur. (*Top left*) Y fracture. (*Bottom right*) T fracture. (*Top right*) Downward movement of the femur into the intercondylar fracture site separating the two condyles.

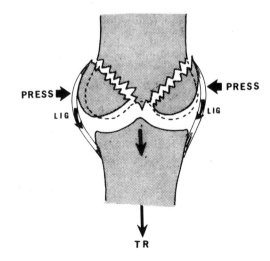

Figure 7–5. Principles of management of intercondylar femoral fracture. Traction (TR) elongates the femur by pulling on the collateral ligaments (LIG) attached to the condyles, bringing them distally where lateral and medial pressure (PRESS), manually or by clamp, will approximate the fragments and reduce the fracture in order to allow casting.

reduction is often necessary to gain proper reduction and to maintain the reduction. The technique will not be detailed. Several types of internal fixation are shown in Figure 7–6.

Condylar Fractures

Condylar fractures are caused by a direct blow, as are supracondylar and intercondylar fractures, but usually of a different type. Whereas supracondylar and *Y* or *T* intercondylar fractures are often caused by direct linear force, fracture of a condyle occurs from a severe varus or valgus force (Fig. 7–7). The fracture line can be in various planes but usually is vertical and in the sagittal plane. The ligaments of the involved side usually prevent marked displacement, but the ligaments of the opposite side and the cruciate ligaments are often damaged.

Management of these fractures depends exclusively on the exact repositioning of the displaced fragment(s) in order to regain continuity of the femoral surface and proper alignment with its opposing tibial surface. Closed

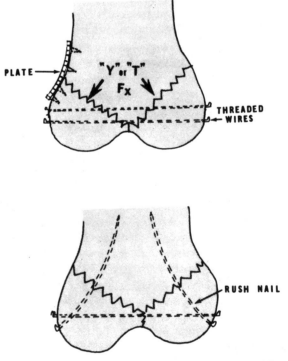

Figure 7–6. Internal fixation methods of supracondylar fractures of the distal femur.

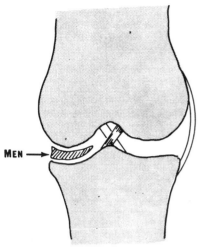

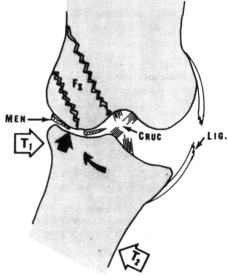

Figure 7–7. Condylar fracture from severe valgus (varus) stress. (*Top*) Normal joint anatomy. (*Bottom*) Force applied to the knee joint (T_1) or laterally to the tibia (T_2) can cause fracture of that condyle (Fx), tear of the opposite ligament (LIG), tear of either or both of the cruciate ligaments (CRUC), and compression of the meniscus (MEN).

reduction by traction and manipulation may succeed. Open reduction, using internal fixation of the fragments and repair of the involved ligaments, is often required. Status of the ligaments must be ascertained in addition to careful documentation of the exact site and extent of the fractured condyle.

Separation of the Distal Epiphysis

This occurrence may be the result of trauma and will be mentioned only briefly here. The condition occurs usually in boys between the ages of 8 and 14 years, usually from a direct blow. Several types are shown in Figure 7–8.

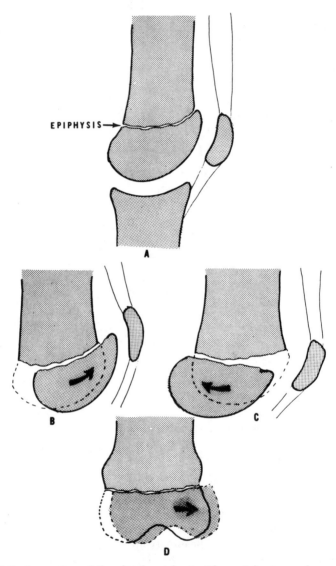

Figure 7–8. Separation of the distal epiphysis. The epiphysis can be separated, depending on the direction of the force. (*A*) The normal epiphysis. (*B*) The epiphysis is tilted forward. (*C*) The rarer type in which the epiphysis is tilted backward. (*D*) The epiphysis may be displaced medially or laterally also.

FRACTURES OF PROXIMAL END OF TIBIA

The upper end of the tibia comprises two large condyles separated by a relatively weak bony span (Fig. 7–9). This fact predisposes the tibial plateau to a high incidence of fractures. The history depicts the exact mechanism of the trauma causing the fracture, usually direct violence linear to the tibia or violent lateral stresses causing forceful abduction or adduction of the knee. The former is exemplified by landing on one's feet following a hard fall; the latter is exemplified by being struck from the side as often happens in an athletic injury or after being hit by a moving vehicle.

The lateral condyle is fractured more frequently than the medial and is associated with injury to the medial ligamentous structures and the cruciate ligaments. The extent of downward or lateral displacement or both is related to the force of the injury. The lateral meniscus may be crushed, forced within the comminution, or forced into the knee joint medially (Fig. 7–10). Severe adduction force on the tibia (lateral force upon the knee joint) may cause fracture of the medial condyle, tearing of the lateral collateral ligaments, and crushing of the medial meniscus.

A direct blow, such as a fall on extended legs, can cause vertical fracture of the tibial plateau in a *Y* or *T* fracture (Fig. 7–11). The ligaments may remain intact or be individually or singly injured. The center fragment may project into the fracture site and cause varying degrees of deformity. Effusion of the joint with blood is usual as these fractures are intra-articular in nature.

Management demands complete evaluation of the mechanism of frac-

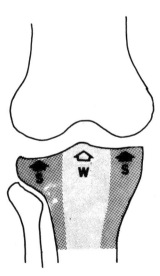

Figure 7–9. Tibial condyles: stress plates. The upper end of the tibia is composed of two condyles: strong cortical bone (S) separated by a weaker bone span (W).

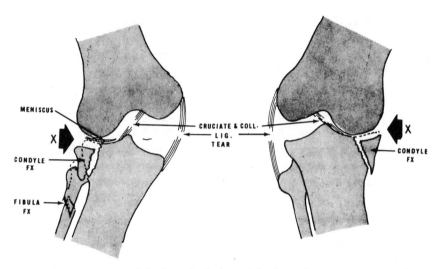

Figure 7–10. Fracture of the lateral tibial condyle. Lateral stress or uneven direct force can cause depressed fracture of the lateral condyle, crushed lateral meniscus, tear of cruciate ligaments, and tear of the medial collateral ligaments.

ture, relationship of the residual fragments, ligamentous injury, and the sequelae of soft tissue injuries. The aim of treatment is to restore the articular surfaces to their anatomic relationships, that is, restoration of the tibial plateau articular surface, proper relationship to the femoral condyles, restoration of ligamentous integrity, evacuation of any intra-articular debris, and restoration of quadriceps strength.

Management of fracture of the lateral tibial condyle begins with aspiration of hemarthrosis. If there is no displacement, start active quadri-

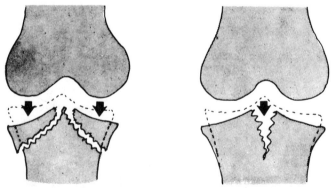

Figure 7–11. Direct trauma to the tibial plateau. Direct trauma, such as a fall on extended legs, can cause a Y or T fracture of the plateau.

ceps exercises after application of a snug-fitting *unpadded* plaster cast with the knee in full extension. In 2 weeks a new plaster is applied, which remains an additional 2 weeks, when flexion exercises are begun. Weight bearing is usually permitted in 10 to 12 weeks, although crutch ambulation without weight bearing is started much sooner.

If the lateral fragment is separated and depressed after the joint is aspirated, traction along the line of the tibia is applied (Fig. 7–12) with simultaneous lateral traction applied by a large bandage passing about the medial aspect of the knee to cause varus of the knee. This last maneuver causes the lateral collateral ligament to pull up on the tibial fragment and reduce the separation. Direct pressure by the surgeon on the fragment will further reduce the depression. A compression clamp may be used by an experienced surgeon. Medial depressed tibial fractures are treated in a similar manner with the forces applied in the opposite transverse direction to cause knee *valgus*.

After reduction, the leg is casted and exercises begun as stated. The cast is kept on for 8 weeks with weight bearing possible in 10 to 12 weeks, preferably *without* a knee brace if the quadriceps is sufficiently strong.

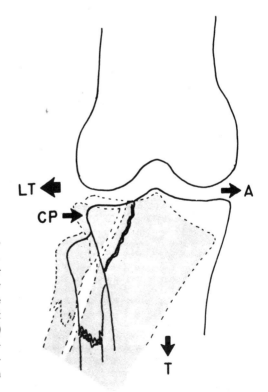

Figure 7–12. Principles of treatment of tibial plateau fracture. Aspirate (A) the hemarthrosis or effusion; apply traction (T); apply lateral traction (LT) to cause varus and open the lateral aspect of the joint; compression (CP) against fragment to reduce fracture, which can be done manually or with a clamp. Cast with snug plaster.

In a severely comminuted fracture, the fragments may be avascular and result in aseptic necrosis. The fragments may wedge the separated fragments and prevent close opposition. If the fragments remain separated and the surface margin irregular, degenerative arthritis, far more severe than normally expected, may result. Tears in the cartilage become filled with fibrous tissue and may create an adequate weight-bearing surface with full range of motion.

If immediate reduction is not attainable, prolonged traction in a Bohler-Braun splint using 10 to 12 lb of traction may be beneficial for reduction. If closed reduction is not possible, open reduction with internal fixation after reduction may be necessary. These indications and techniques are well documented in the orthopedic literature.

FRACTURES OF THE PATELLA

Because the patella is exposed, it is a frequent site of fractures. It is easy to suspect that trauma has occurred because of the pain, swelling, dislocation, tenderness, and functional impairment. The history may include a direct blow from an object or from a fall. The flexed knee, particularly the patella, is susceptible to injuries in car accidents.

The examination should be compatible with the suggestive history. There is local tenderness and often swelling and discoloration. The contour of the injured patella, as compared to the normal patella, is deformed. If fragmentation has occurred, it can often be manually palpated. X-ray films are diagnostic for the presence, site, extent, and continuity of the injury.

Conservative treatment or surgery may be warranted. If there is no separation of the fragments and therefore normal contour, conservative treatment of the fracture can be considered. The knee can be placed in a posterior mold and splinted in full extension. Excessive effusion and especially hemarthrosis should be aspirated under sterile conditions. Ice applied for 20 minutes every hour decreases further effusion or its recurrence and diminishes pain. TENS may be of value if there is a great deal of pain.

Isometric quadriceps contraction exercises should be initiated within a few days to avoid or minimize the rapid onset of atrophy that results from avoiding the use of the knee because of pain and/or effusion. Electrical stimulation to the quadriceps may initiate contraction that prevents atrophy. Electrical stimulation initiates contraction when the muscle is paretic from pain and/or effusion.

A cast may be applied after effusion has decreased, but local pressure on the patella must be avoided. Where there is the reason to remove and view the underlying tissues, a bivalve cast is best. However, a Velcro-strapped splint with a patellar cutout is the most desirable type of immobilization.

The patella should be conserved if at all possible in spite of the many statements that it is an unnecessary bone. If the fragments are in good opposition, no further direct care is needed; the injury will heal in time. If there are a few large fragments, they can be openly reduced and wired. Only if there is severe fragmentation beyond repair and reconstruction should a patellectomy be considered.

The principles of surgery are essentially:

1. Repositioning and fixing the fragments in place
2. Removal of all the smaller fragments, allowing the major fragment to remain
3. Total patellectomy
4. Replacement of the patella with a prosthesis

Repositioning and fixing the fragments in place is often unsuccessful since it is difficult to assure a smooth undersurface for the patella. The irregularity may predispose the knee to degenerative arthritis and abrasion of the femoral condyles. The quadriceps pulling on the fragments may prevent good healing, and there is little osteogenesis of the patella. Prosthetics are being perfected, and orthopedic surgeons are learning to use them.

CAUSALGIA AND OTHER REFLEX SYMPATHETIC DYSTROPHIES

Causalgia

Causalgia involves the lower extremities somewhat less frequently than it does the upper extremities. This condition is frequently seen in wartime, but with the increasing incidence of warlike injuries in civilian life and automobile and motorcycle accidents, it is appearing more frequently in peacetime.

Conservative and surgical treatments of injuries in the vicinity of the knee often result in reflex sympathetic dystrophy (RSD) in the lower extremity, which may be overlooked. The most frequent cause of RSD in the lower extremity is iatrogenic, that is, from surgical interventions, tight casts, and injuries near or of nerves of the lower extremity. RSD in the absence of causalgia is often misdiagnosed and mistreated with severe disabling sequelae.

Reflex Sympathetic Dystrophy

Reflex sympathetic dystrophy now encompasses many neuromuscular vasomotor disabling conditions of both lower and upper extremities. This condition, aptly termed a syndrome, is known to follow virtually any form of local injury, whether major or minor. The condition, originally called "causalgia," implied *burning pain* with associated neurovascular symptomatology. This syndrome is broken down into major and minor forms; the minor form is not associated with pain. Delineating the condition in this way helps physicians to more readily recognize it early and treat it properly.

Bonica[2] divided RSD into the major and minor subdivisions (Table 7–1). It is apparent that any trauma can be implicated for the minor dystrophies, including an incident that is so minor that it is difficult to remember.

Both major and minor RSD occur in the upper extremity; therefore, this syndrome is discussed in *Shoulder Pain.*[3] Since RSD is a major complication of any painful or painless upper extremity impairment, the physician must consider RSD for any complaint of the arm.

Burning pain and associated symptomatology following a peripheral nerve injury was noted by Paré[4] in the 16th century. It reached prominence during the U.S. Civil War when it was described by Mitchell, Morehouse, and Keen.[5] They described the condition in wounded soldiers who developed a burning pain following peripheral nerve injury, usually from a gunshot wound. The term "causalgia" was employed for describing the burning character of the pain. This condition is currently classified as a major reflex sympathetic dystrophy.

Many clinicians followed with descriptive discussions of this condition. Letievant[6] ascribed a neurological cause to this condition. Sudeck[7] published a classic description of the radiological characteristics of bone osteoporosis following trauma with subsequent RSD. Leriche[8] described the condition as a sequela of trauma to the sympathetic nervous system. As a result, peripheral sympathectomy became a favored and successful treatment for RSD. RSD was largely forgotten until World War II, when numerous cases were reported and the clinical condition was revived.

Numerous terms for this condition have been used in the literature, such as algodystrophy, sympathalgia, neurovascular reflex sympathetic dystrophy, traumatic angiospasm, traumatic vasospasm, Sudeck atrophy, posttraumatic osteoporosis, posttraumatic painful osteoporosis, and shoul-

Table 7–1. REFLEX SYMPATHETIC DYSTROPHY

Major	Minor
Causalgia	Shoulder-hand-finger syndrome
Thalamic syndrome	Postmyocardial infarct
Phantom limb	Postcerebrovascular attack
	Postinjection*
	Postfracture, cast, or splint*
	Postoveruse syndrome*

*Indicates RSD with knee involvement.

der-hand-finger syndrome. Since the pain persists, often even after the initial trauma subsides, and since pain is considered to reside in the peripheral nervous system via the sympathetic nerve fibers, the persistent pain has been labeled sympathetic-maintained pain (SMP). When there is less evidence of sympathetic nervous system involvement, then the persistent pain has been labeled sympathetic-independent pain (SIP).[9]

All the above references allude to the clinical manifestations of:

1. Persistent pain, which was described in various ways but frequently had a burning or similar quality
2. Vasomotor changes, manifested as hyperthermia and often followed by coldness
3. A subcutaneous edema that rapidly becomes nonpitting
4. Sensory changes, at first hyperesthesia and later hypoesthesia
5. Ultimately trophic changes such as atrophy of the skin, muscle, and bone,[10] causing functional impairment, significant osteoporosis, and atrophic osteoarthrosis[11]

Causalgia has been defined by the International Association for the Study of Pain (IASP) as "a syndrome of sustained burning pain after traumatic nerve lesion combined with vasomotor and sudomotor dysfunction and later trophic changes."[12] The RSD syndrome has been expanded to include many conditions that lack burning pain yet have all the vasomotor and sudomotor symptomatology and other findings. This would conform to the definition of SID pain advocated by Roberts.[8] The basic mechanisms, pathophysiology, and symptomatology[12] are so similar in the two forms of RSD as to justify the diagnostic term and therapies.

Close scrutiny of the words that comprise the term "RSD" clearly clarifies this disease entity. "Dystrophy" indicates a wasting of the muscular and bony tissues of a region, abnormal growth of the nails of the affected extremity, and hyperkeratosis of the skin. "Sympathetic" indicates vasomotor and sudomotor changes such as inappropriate sweating, coldness, and color changes of the extremity from vasoconstriction or vasodilation. "Reflex" indicates that the signs emanate from the sympathetic nervous system distribution of the extremity. Another confirmatory diagnostic fact of RSD is its beneficial response to sympathetic interruption.

In major RSD (causalgia) the onset of pain is either immediate or occurs within a brief period of time, whereas in minor RSD there may be a delay of onset of pain of from several days to months. To qualify as being RSD, the character of the pain must be of a burning quality. The site of the symptoms seen in this syndrome is distal in the extremity, be it upper shoulder-hand-finger or lower knee-ankle-foot-toes.

Various mechanisms have been postulated, such as the one proposed by Mitchell, Morehouse, and Keen[5] that there is "an inexplicable reflex in the spinal cord centers felt in remote regions outside the distribution of the wounded nerve." This definition has been modified by the author, but the idea is retained. A more recent hypothesis has been offered by Devor,[14] who postulates that the injury damages or transects the involved nerve. This appealing theory requires an understanding of the structure of nerve axons and of axoplasmic transport. The hypothesis is exemplified in Figure 7–13 (modified from Ochs[15]).

Neuronal function is now considered to be axonal transport of protein and other materials needed by the tissues supplied by the nerve. Sensory impulses are also similarly carried by axonal transport.

The neuron cell body is the site of a high level of protein synthesis, and these proteins are transported along the length of the nerve fiber via the axonal microtubules and neurofilaments. This transport mechanism has been shown to be very dependent on adequate blood suppply. Pressure on the nerve axon and/or its blood flow will impair axonal transport. The identity of the components of the proteins of the peripheral nerve also affect axonal impairment.[16]

After a nerve is constricted, the fibers may show collateral branching.[17,18] During recovery of the injured nerve, the exposed regenerating surface of the axon undergoes a more than normal accumulation of alpha-

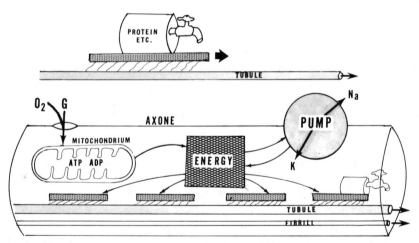

Figure 7–13. Axoplasmic neural transport, a theory. The flow of protein and other derivatives begins with entry of glucose (G) into the fiber. Glycolysis and phosphorylation occurs (O_2) in the mitochondria through metabolism of adenosine-triphosphate (ATP) which creates the energy to the sodium pump. This pump regulates balance of sodium (Na) and potassium (K) and determines nerve activity.

The transport filaments (F) move along the axon by oscillation and carry the nutritive protein elements along the nerve pathway. (Data from Ochs: Axoplasmic transport—A basis for neural pathology.)

adrenergic receptors, which results in abnormal electrical properties. These excessive, and possibly abnormal, receptors become ectopic pacemakers that lead to spontaneous depolarization. Being numerous and excessive, the affected nerves bombard the central nervous system and interfere with normal processing of CNS sensory information. The central nervous system, which is already in a state of hyperactivity and hyperreceptivity from previous bombardment by unmyelinated nerve fiber impulses, is now bombarded by distal adrenaline[18] impulses from new branchings of nerve fibers[13] (Fig. 7–14). The peripheral stimuli originate because of abnormal chemosensitivity and mechanosensitivity of the neurons and not as a result of other physiological stimuli.

The aberrant sensory processing of this barrage by the CNS produces a sensation of pain (paresthesia). The altered sympathetic reflexes produce the somatic characteristics of RSD (Fig. 7–15).

There are other theories that involve the peripheral nervous system and do not include the central nervous system. One theory is that at the site of the nerve injury a synapse between efferent sympathetic fibers and afferent pain fibers "short circuits" the sensory information.[19] This hypothesis has been refuted because it does not explain why a sympathetic nerve block distal to the lesion occurs. There is another hypothesis[21] which invokes the liberation of algogenic substances at the involved areas of trauma which produce local hyperalgesia which in turn causes further local noxious vasomotor substances.

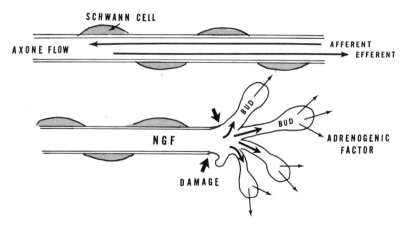

Figure 7–14. Axonal outgrowths forming a neuroma (schematic). After a nerve injury with compression or partial to total severence, the nerve growth factor (NGF) stimulates the nerve to advance distally and form "buds" which create more endings than the normal nerve shown in the upper drawing.

By virtue of the greater secretion of adrenogenic factors from these additional buds, the nerve becomes more sensitive to adrenogenic agonists and transmits more potential pain fiber impulses to the spinal cord.

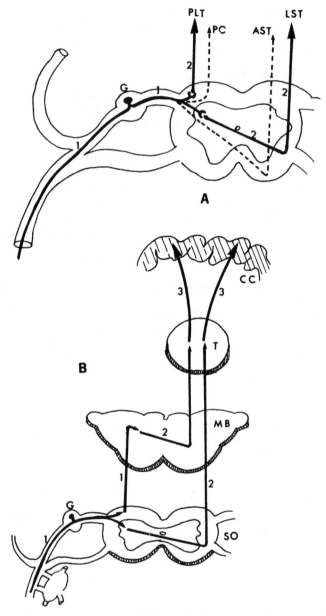

Figure 7–15. Neuronal pathways of pain. (A) The course of sensory fibers in a segmental nerve with its ganglion in the dorsal root (G). Upon entrance into the cord, the fibers ascend on the same side in the posterior lateral tract (PLT) and decussate to cross into the lateral spinothalamic tract; 2 indicates secondary neurons. The posterior column (PC) transmits position sense; anterior spinal thalamic tract (AST) conveys tactile sensation. (B) 1 = first-stage neurons to the cord; 2 = second-stage neurons through the midbrain (MB) into the thalamus (T); 3 = third-stage neurons, the thalamocortical pathways to the cerebral cortex (CC).

Of the numerous mechanisms that involve the CNS, the concept of bombardment of the dorsal horn cells in laminae IV to VI by peripheral nociceptor substances is widely accepted (Fig. 7–16).

As stated by Rizzi, Visentin, and Mazzetti,[21] it is not clear why causalgia most often occurs with a "partial" nerve lesion rather than a complete lesion, especially because it is observed so infrequently in partial nerve lesions.

The psychological state of the individual at the time of injury has also been postulated to be a significant factor.[22,23] More research is needed to ascertain the neural-psychological-humoral susceptibility of individuals under extreme anxiety that predisposes patients with trauma to develop causalgic RSD.

A hypothesis[24] has recently been advanced to explain why many cases of RSD occur after a relatively minor trauma or why pain and other somatic symptoms are exacerbated by emotional stress. Pre-existing anxiety and stress are postulated to increase release of norepinephrine, which increases arteriolar hyperactivity. The resultant vasospasm and ischemia, and the release of nociceptors on neural tissues already bathed by excessive norepinephrine from the anxiety and stress, result in RSD.

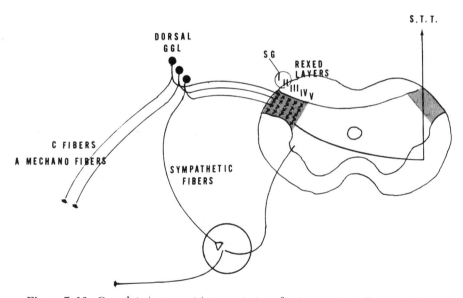

Figure 7–16. Causalgic (autonomic) transmission of pain sensation. Trauma irritates somatic afferent C-fibers, A-mechanofibers, and sympathetic fibers, whose impulses proceed to the dorsal column of the cord. There is a cord interneuron connection that transmits efferent impulses via the autonomic system to the periphery, which sensitizes the skin to mechanical (light touch) input.

At the cord, the afferent fibers initiate neuronal activity in the Rexed layers of the dorsal column. The Rexed layers I and II are the substantia gelatinosa. (Modified from Roberts, WS: A hypothesis on the physiological basis for causalgia and related pains. Pain 24:297, 1986.)

Local and referred pain are often aggravated by minor, unrelated, and reasonably innocuous stimuli that are transmitted to the central nervous system via mechanoreceptors. These receptors and their afferent fibers normally do not transmit pain, but in this condition, SMP, they enhance the pain. This concept is illustrated in Figure 7–17.

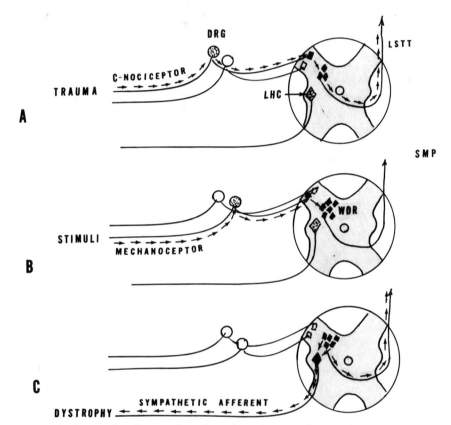

Figure 7–17. Postulated neurophysiological mechanism of sympathetic-maintained pain (SMP). The transmission via C-nociceptor fibers (A) of impulses from the peripheral tissues that have been traumatized and created peripheral nociceptor chemicals (see details in text). These impulses pass through the dorsal root ganglion (DRG) to activate the gray matter of the cord in the Rexed layers. When sensitized, they are termed *wise dynamic range neurons* (WDR). The WDR, becoming very irritated, receive impulses from the periphery via the A-mechanoreceptor fibers, (B) which normally transmit sensations of touch, vibration, temperature, etc. When the periphery is stimulated (skin touch, pressure, or joint movement), these impulses enhance and maintain the irritability of the WDR. The impulses from the WDR continue cephalad through the lateral spinal thalamic tracts (LSTT) to the thalamic centers with resultant continued pain. The WDR impulses irritate the lateral horn cells (LHC), which generate sympathetic impulses that innervate the peripheral tissues resulting in the symptoms and findings of dystrophy (C).

Nerve action potentials following the trauma are transmitted through C-nociceptive fibers to the dorsal root ganglion and then to the spinal cord in the region of the dorsal horn (Rexed layers). They bombard that region, forming a hypersensitive set of neurons (termed "wide dynamic range neurons," or WDR, by Roberts[20]). The WDR can then be bombarded by impulses via the mechanoreceptors from, for example, the skin, muscles, tendons, and ligaments that travel via A-mechanofibers of myelinated nerves. These impulses impinge on the already hypersensitive cord regions, that is, the WDR, which can "spill" over or influence the proximal nerve cells (lateral horn) of the autonomic (sympathetic) nerves. This indicates how innocuous unrelated touch, pressure, or movement can intensify the pain even though mechanoreceptors, not nociceptors, are involved. These impulses then travel distally (efferent) to the periphery, causing vasomotor reactions as well as stimulating sympathetic nervous system pain sensations.

The evolving vasomotor changes of the dystrophy are thus explained. The theory also explains the basis of sympathetic afferent impulses initiating the cycle, which is then enhanced by mechanoreceptor irritants such as touch, stretch, and passive and active motion.

In the symptomatic lower extremity RSD lesions, which eventually develop into minor or major RSD, the etiology may remain unknown, but its occurrence demands attention, both diagnostic and therapeutic, to minimize the disabling sequelae.

Reflex Sympathetic Dystrophy in the Lower Extremity

Posttraumatic lower extremity injuries are not classified as causalgia unless, by definition, a partial nerve lesion has occurred. In conditions such as fractures, dislocations, and poststroke hemiparetic lower extremity lesions, a nerve lesion is not required for RSD to develop. The minor RSD lesion of knee-foot-ankle syndrome, regardless of the etiology, usually does not have a partial nerve lesion or develop a painful causalgia. However, all the sequelae of RSD do develop.

Leg-Foot-Ankle RSD Syndrome

In this condition there is dysfunction of the sympathetic nervous system but from a different physiological basis and from a different etiological entity. As a rule this RSD has a mechanical basis, that is, there is nerve pressure and a neurovascular response.

The somatic nerve supply to the lower extremity (Figs. 7–18 and 7–19) is accompanied by sympathetic nerves. The normal circulation of the lower extremity can be simplistically divided into arterial and venous components, both of which have a mechanical component.

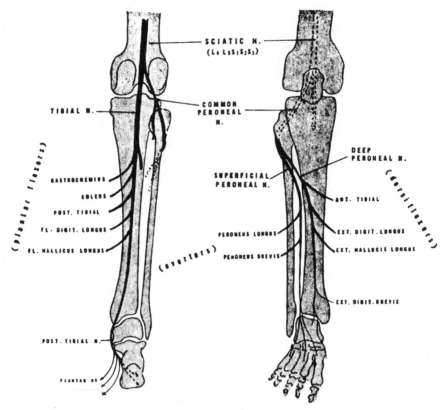

Figure 7–18. Innervation of the leg and foot. The sciatic nerve divides at the popliteal angle to form the tibial nerve and the common peroneal nerve.

1. The arterial component is the cardiac *pumping* action, the major arterial tone, the constriction-relaxation cycle, and the gravitational forces that propel the arterial blood flow to the distal portions of the upper extremities. Blood flows via the major arteries, into the arterioles, and then into the capillaries, where there is diffusion into the tissues.

2. The blood is circulated back to the heart and lungs via the venous and lymphatic channels by virtue of *pump* action. The muscles of the calf and anterior compartment literally pump the blood proximally with the assistance of gravity. The leg must frequently be held above heart level for gravity to be effective. The lower leg muscles thus act as a pump in this activity. The thigh, knee, and ankle muscles move the leg, ankle, and foot in every direction. In addition to pumping the venous blood and lymphatic fluid toward the heart, this is aided by elevating the lower extremity above heart level (Fig. 7–20).

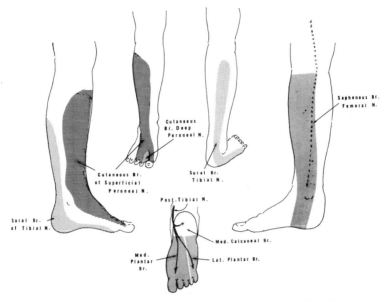

Figure 7–19. Sensory patterns of peripheral nerves of the leg.

Repeated contraction and relaxation of the leg muscles pump the blood and lymphatic fluid proximally. Failure of either of these pumps to function adequately may lead to a painful and disabling condition termed leg-foot-ankle (LFA) syndrome. Loss of alternating flexion and extension in the ankle eliminates the distal pump. As is well known, a fracture dislocation of the knee with or without a cast may initiate this condition.

Pain from this syndrome is described as an "ache," deep discomfort, tenderness, painful movement, or even mild "burning." Pain usually does not occur initially or necessarily early in this process; it may only be noted several days to weeks after onset. Most often there are impairments of function other than pain, which is why in many cases the condition is not diagnosed early.

Mechanism. The sequela of the leg-foot-ankle syndrome from whatever initial condition is that the muscular pump does not function. Inadequate hip and knee motion impairs the upper pump action, and there is a decrease in venous lymphatic flow.

Factors that may initiate limited motion are:

1. Meniscus tears
2. Ligamentous tears, collateral or cruciate
3. Fracture and dislocation of the bones of and adjacent to the knee joint

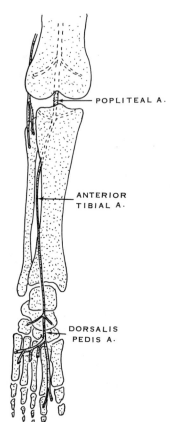

Figure 7–20. Blood supply to the lower extremity.

4. Posthemiplegic knee-foot-ankle impairment
5. Postoperative casting
6. Soft tissue surgical procedures

Diagnosis. The knee and/or ankle may become "stiff," that is, there is limited passive and active range of motion. The cause of this limitation must be discerned and addressed. Most of these causes have been discussed previously and will not be repeated here, but in addition to the many knee problems, the following must also be considered:

1. Systemic paresis such as Guillain-Barré syndrome and poliomyelitis
2. Spinal cord injury with paraplegia or quadriplegia
3. Inappropriate immobilization from a cast or a sustained position

The onset of the LFA syndrome is first noted in the foot, where subtle edema appears on the dorsum and in the toes. The skin becomes "shiny," smooth, and pale. At first pitting may be elicited, but the degree of pitting is usually so minimal that it may escape attention.

Flexion of the full ankle plantar and dorsum as well as the active and passive range of motion of the toes is decreased. Evaluation requires careful attention since the degree of limitation is so minimal that it must be compared to the opposite foot, ankle, and toes or its presence will escape attention. This limited range of motion marks the subtle beginning of the loss of the distal pump. Movement of the toes and the ankle becomes limited as a result of the edema under the corresponding tendons.

The skin, which is at first edematous, is also ischemic and becomes thickened and then ultimately atrophic. Clinically hyperhidrosis (from excessive sudomotor activity) occurs early: the foot is moist. It may be either pale or have a slight rubor. The color change depends on whether there is vasodilation or vasoconstriction (from impaired vasomotor tone). The foot is thus moist, pale, and either cold or warm. When compared with the normal foot, the vasomotor and sudomotor abnormalities are noted early in the condition.

Although in RSD the affected skin is more often cold (vasoconstriction) than warm (vasodilation), there is *increased* blood flow in the subcutaneous tissues,[25] muscles,[26] and bones.[27] This increased blood flow to the bone may account for the increased activity noted in radioactive bone scans in RSD. The increased deeper blood flow may also initiate a transient arteriovenous shunt with decreased superficial blood flow, hence the ultimate dystrophy.

The hair follicles and nails also thicken (hypertrichosis) from excessive sudomotor activity. All these sudomotor and vasomotor changes are, at first, subtle, but gradually they become progressively more pronounced. The stage at which they are discovered and treatment started determines the correctability and reversibility of the structural changes.

The stages of LFA syndrome are as follows:

Stage 1. Vasomotor signs of hyperhidrosis with edema. The following are also found:

- Limited range of motion (with or without pain) of the toes and ankle.
- Swelling of the dorsum of the foot and ankle, and pitting is observed.
- Shiny and dry or moist skin.
- Limited range of motion of the foot and ankle and flexion of the toe.
- Pain on flexing the ankle dorsum and plantar

Stage 2. The most significant change in the edema is that it is "firmer" and cannot be dimpled by pressure. The following are also found:

• The foot and ankle pain may subside, and there may be a slight increase in the active and passive range of motion.
• Edema of the foot appears to subside, and there is less pitting
• The skin is less elastic, and it becomes less sensitive
• The toes have become stiffer
• The nails and hairs have become coarser
• Osteoporosis becomes evident on x-ray films

Stage 3. The following are found:

• There is progressive atrophy of the bones, skin, and muscles
• There is limited passive range of motion at the ankle and toes
• The nails are brittle and grooved. The hair follicles are large and brittle
• Pain may now be minimal or absent except when passive motion is attempted

X-ray films that reveal bone atrophy (osteoporosis) may be noted as early as stage 1, but usually the atrophy is noted in stage 2. Diagnostic x-ray films should always include the opposite foot for comparison since early changes are subtle. Methods for determining bone density that differentiate and grade the degree of osteoporosis have been developed, but they are academic. It must be stated that the initial diagnosis *must not be made on finding bone density changes in foot x-rays* since by then stage 3 has begun.

During the progression of the LFA syndrome there are ultimately atrophic articular changes. Because of the ischemia that results from vasomotor abnormality, the cartilage of the tarsal, metatarsal, and phalangeal bones impairs the circulation in the joints, producing atrophic arthritis. Neither passive nor active motion is possible. There is no pain, but the ankle, foot, and toes also do not function.

Stages 1 and 2 are considered functionally reversible. Stage 3 has many irreversible structural changes that make functional recovery limited, if at all feasible.

A timely diagnosis is to suspect when subtle skin changes of the foot occur in any of the following conditions of the lower extremity:

1. An ankle "problem" where there is pain and limited motion
2. Pain or limited motion of the foot
3. Pain and limited motion of the digits of the hand
4. Trauma to the lower extremity such as surgery, injection, or a sprain or strain
5. A systemic condition with referred pain to the lower extremity

Treatment. Treatment of reflex sympathetic dystrophy varies only slightly depending on whether there is causalgic pain, because the tissue changes of dystrophy present the major residual disabling factors. Causalgic pain must be immediately and forcefully treated by sympathetic vasomotor intervention since the syndrome cannot be remedied or even moderated without relief of pain. Relief of the causalgic pain also indicates that the intervention is beginning to reverse the dystrophic tissue changes.

Treatment of the sequelae of RSD must be initiated simultaneously and as energetically as the treatment of causalgia. To relieve the pain but have the tissue changes progress from stage 2 to stage 3 does not benefit the patient.

Interruption of sympathetic hyperactivity in the lower extremity can be initiated by a chemical blocking agent administered via the caudal or epidural route. Benefit from a chemical sympathetic nervous system blocker becomes both diagnostic and therapeutic. Verification of vasomotor change and relief of pain indicates that the sympathetic nervous system is hyperactive as well as permitting the patient to accept and undergo active therapy aimed at the tissues of the lower extremity.

A series of epidural blocks should be considered and undertaken so long as they produce satisfactory results. A series of four blocks is feasible with the consideration of installation of an epidural catheter and/or the administration of other medications either epidurally, intravenously, intra-arterially, or even via a sympathectomy.[3]

Sympathetic intervention can be termed "good" if:

1. One block gives total relief.
2. One block gives significant relief of pain.
3. After a beneficial first block, subsequent blocks give further significant relief.

It is termed "poor" if:

1. The first block has a beneficial effect, but each subsequent block is less effective or totally ineffective.
2. The initial benefit of the block wears off after the anesthetic (from the anesthesia added for instillation) is gone. This fact questions whether the relief is a result of steroidal intervention in the sympathetic nervous system or merely temporary anesthesia.

If no benefit is gained from repeated chemical sympathetic nervous system interventions, then there is a good indication that there will be little benefit from surgical intervention of the sympathetic nervous system.

Oral or intramuscular steroids have been advocated and found benefi-

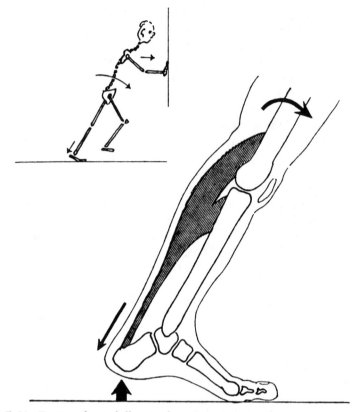

Figure 7–21. Testing the Achilles tendon elongation in the erect position. The patient stands away from the wall and leans against it. The leg to be tested remains behind with the knee extended and the heel against the floor. The other leg is brought forward, the knee bent, and the foot elevated. The Achilles tendon is stretched as the body leans forward. The heel will rise from the floor if the Achilles is shortened, and characteristic pain can be reproduced. This movement may also be used as an exercise to stretch the heel cord.

cial. As with any prescribed medication, the undesirable side effects must be known and weighed against the possible benefits. The dosage and duration of administration must be carefully monitored.

Intravenous injections of guanethidine[28] into the affected extremity have been advocated. The injection is administered into the extremity restricted by appropriate application of a blood pressure cuff.

In the presence of persistent pain, the use of transcutaneous electric nerve stimulus (TENS) is worth trying. If after a reasonable period of time, the benefit is minimal, further use is considered worthless. It is mandatory that, before abandoning TENS, the placement of the electrodes, dosage, and current be confirmed as correct.[29,30]

Every mode of treatment must be tried in the management of RSD of the lower extremity, including:

1. Local application of ice alternating with a moist heat pack to the extremity for periods of 20 minutes q.i.d.

2. Passive and active range of motion exercises of the knee, ankle, foot, and toes.

3. Active resisted exercises to regain and maintain strength and endurance of the quadriceps, gastrocnemius, and anterior tibialis, invertors, and evertors, as well as all the muscles of the toes (Fig. 7–21).

4. Frequent elevation of the legs during the day for lengthy periods of time.

5. Removal of edema by vasoconstrictive stockings with or without a daily massage.

6. Electrical stimulation at the motor points of the affected muscles. This can initiate active contraction when there is significant weakness, early atrophy, and inability to exercise because of pain.

7. Daily passive mobilization of every joint of the foot and ankle by a therapist and/or a trained member of the family.

8. Orthotics within the shoe to permit ambulation with minimal pain by decreasing the effects of pressure points (Figs. 7–22, 7–23, and 7–24).

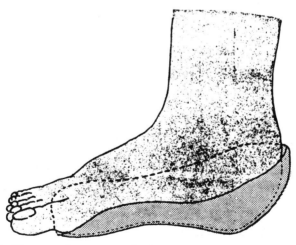

Figure 7–22. The UC-BL shoe insert. The laminated fiberglass insert shell is molded over a plaster mold of the foot. It fits snugly into the shoe. The heel is held in a neutral position and the forefoot held in an adducted supinated position.

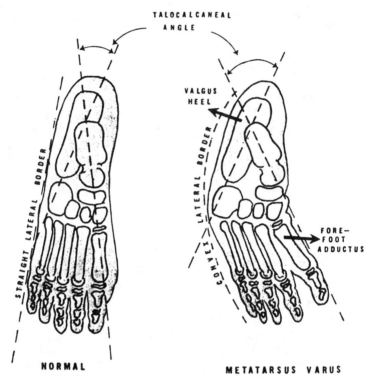

Figure 7–23. Components of metatarsus varus compared to the normal foot. Metatarsus varus has an adducted forefoot and a valgus heel. The lateral margin of the foot is convex with the apex at the base of the fifth metatarsal. The talus is medially and anteriorly displaced in relationship to the calcaneus, thus increasing the talo calcaneal angle.

Psychiatric Aspects of RSD

The full psychiatric implications of reflex sympathetic dystrophy are beyond the scope of this text. However, the subject of RSD cannot be dismissed without consideration of this subject.

White and Sweet[30] suggested that because emotional factors are so prevalent in this condition, a placebo diagnostic test should be performed before continuing with sympathetic nerve blockers or significant surgical intervention. If relief is obtained after a local anesthetic block but not after a sterile saline injection, then a therapeutic block can be considered.

The medical literature frequently states that individuals with a *periarthritic personality* or a *type A personality* are prone to develop RSD. The question of an emotional component has been alluded to[18] and raises the question as to whether RSD is purely psychogenic, hysterical, or even malingering. With the current limited knowledge of the psychological

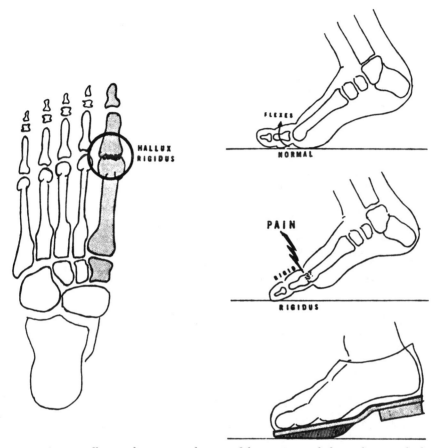

Figure 7–24. Hallux rigidus. Due to damage of the metatarsophalangeal joint, which becomes rigid, the toe will not flex on toe-off of the gait, and pain can occur at each step. Treatment consists of preventing stress on the rigid toe by placing a steel plate in the shoe sole to prevent bending and a rocker bar to permit pain-free gait.

aspects of many painful states, only consideration without verification can be ascertained.

In active RSD, the emotional state of the patient whether causative or merely contributory must be taken into consideration. Anxiety must be allayed, and depression must be recognized and addressed with counseling, medication, and, where it is warranted, psychiatric intervention.

REFERENCES

1. Olebud, S: Operative treatment of supracondylar-condylar fractures of the femur. J Bone Joint Surg 54A:1015, 1972.

2. Bonica, JJ: Causalgia and other reflex sympathetic dystrophies. In Bonica, JJ, Liebeskind, JC, and Albe-Fessard, D (eds): Research and Therapy, Vol. 3. Raven Press, New York, 1979, p 141.

3. Cailliet, R: Shoulder pain. FA Davis, Philadelphia, 1991, p 227.

4. Paré, A: Les oeuvres d'abrose paré. 2:115, 1840.

5. Mitchell, SW, Morehouse, GR, and Keen, WW: Gunshot Wounds and Other Injuries of Nerves. JB Lippincott, Philadelphia, 1864.

6. Letievant, E: Traite de Section Nerveuses. JB Bailliere et Fils, Paris, 1873.

7. Sudeck, P: Uber die akute entzundlike knockenatrophie. Arch Clin Chir 62:147, 1900.

8. Leriche, R: De la causalgie envisagee comme une nevrite du sympathique et son traitment par la denudation et l'escision des plexus nerveut periarteriees. Presse Med 24:178, 1916.

9. Roberts WJ: A hypothesis on the physiological basis for causalgia and related pains. Pain 24:297, 1986.

10. De Takata, G and Miller, DS: Posttraumatic dystrophy of the extremities. Arch Surg 46:469, 1943.

11. Miller, DS and deTakata, G: Post-traumatic dystrophy of the extremities (Sudeck's atrophy). Surg Gynec Obst 75:538, 1943.

12. Merskey, H: Classification of chronic pain: Description of chronic pain syndromes and definitions of pain terms. Pain (Suppl)3:285, 1986.

13. Tahmouth, AJ: Causalgia: Redefinition as a clinical pain syndrome. Pain 10:187, 1981.

14. Devor, M: Nerve pathophysiology and mechanisms of pain in causalgia. J Autonom Nerv Syst 7:371, 1983.

15. Ochs, S: Axoplasmic transport—a basis for neural pathology. In Dyke, PJ, Thomas, PK, and Lambert, EH (eds): Peripheral Neuropathy. WB Saunders, Philadelphia, 1975, p 213.

16. Garfin, SR, et al: Compressive neuropathy of spinal nerve roots: A mechanical or biological problem? Spine 16: 1991.

17. Perroncito, A: La rigenerazione delle fibre nervose. Boll Soc Med Chir Pavia 4:434, 1905.

18. Shawe, GDH: On the number of branches formed by regenerating nerve fibres. Brit J Surg 42:474, 1955.

19. Doupe, J, et al: Post-traumatic pain and the causalgic syndrome. J Neurol Neurosurg Psychiat 7:33–48.

20. Roberts, WJ: A hypothesis on the physiological basis for causalgia and related pains. Pain 24:297, 1986.

21. Rizzi, R, Visentin, M, and Mazzetti, G: Reflex sympathetic dystrophy. In Benedetti, C, et al (eds): Advances in Pain Research and Therapy, Vol 7. Raven Press, New York, 1984, p 451.

22. Wirth, FP and Rutherford, RB: A civilian experience with causalgia. Arch Surg 100:633, 1970.

23. Owens, JC: Causalgia. Ann Surg 23:636, 1975.

24. Ecker, A: Norepinephrine in reflex sympathetic dystrophy: An hypothesis. Clin J Pain 5:313, 1989.

25. Christensen, K and Henricksen, O: The reflex sympathetic syndrome and experimental study of sympathetic reflex control of subcutaneous blood flow in the hand. Scand J Rheum 12:263, 1983.

26. Sylvest, J, et al: Reflex dystrophy: Resting blood flow and muscle temperature as diagnostic criteria. Scand J Rehab Med 9:25, 1977.

27. Ficat, T, et al: Trans M-A, algodystrophies reflexes post-traumatique. Rev Chir Orthop 59:401, 1973.

28. Hanningthon-Kiff, JG: Relief of causalgia in limbs by regional intravenous guanethidine. Brit Med J 2:367, 1979.

29. Langley, GB, et al: The analgesic effects of transcutaneous electrical nerve stimulation and placebo in chronic pain patients: A double blind non-crossover comparison. Rheum Int 4:119, 1984.

30. Melzack, R, Stillwell, DM, and Fox, EJ: Trigger points and acupuncture points for pain: Correlates and implications. Pain 3:3, 1977.
31. White, JC and Sweet, WH: Pain and the Neurosurgeon: A Forty Year Experience. Charles C Thomas, Springfield, IL, 1969, p 87.
32. Brena, SF and Koch, DL: A "pain estimate" model for quantification and classification of chronic pain states. Anesthesiol Rev 8, 1975.
33. Hendler, N, et al: A comparison between the MMPI and the "Hendler Back Pain Test" for validating the complaint of chronic back pain in men. J Neurol Orthop Med Surg 6:333, 1985.

CHAPTER 8

Congenital and Acquired Deformities of the Knee

In evaluating deformities that involve the knee, the deformity may be considered "congenital" in that it was present at or before birth or "acquired" when its presence became apparent after an otherwise normal birth structure. Deformities may thus be grouped into the following categories:

1. Failure of tissue differentiation, such as failure of cartilage to progress into bone
2. Failure of bony elements to fuse into their expected mature state, for example, the bipartite patella
3. Supernumerary parts
4. Deformity in the bone itself, such as osteogenesis imperfecta or congenital bowing

Bone dysplasia (abnormal development of tissue) is considered to be a congenital variance, although it also has biochemical, hormonal, and metabolic causes. These dystrophies and dysplasias are well documented.[1,2] Most are rare, and few affect only the knee. However, they do involve the knee in conjunction with other general abnormalities in the growing child. *Dysplasia* is described as a disturbance in bone development and is intrinsic to the bone.[2] *Dystrophy* is described as defective bone development caused by *extrinsic* factors such as metabolic or nutritional abnormalities. *Dysostosis* is abnormal development caused by a *defect* in ectodermal or mesenchymal tissue.

In all these conditions, the extremities usually are deformed and shortened causing an abnormal gait. The knee, besides affecting the length of the extremity, may also be involved in the extremity's alignment, that is, varus, valgus, or recurvatum (which denote an inward, outward, and backward bending, respectively, from the midline[3]).

Genu valgum, genu varum, genu recurvatum, and tibial or femoral torsion are the most frequent deformities noted in childhood. They cause parental concern over abnormal gait, stance, or appearance. Although these conditions are usually congenital or familial, they may also be acquired following an injury or may be secondary to systemic disease.

GENU VALGUM

Genu valgum is an angular deformity of the leg, otherwise termed "knock-knee," in which the feet and ankles are markedly separated when the knees are in contact (Fig. 8–1). This condition is frequently noted in childhood, and there appears to be a family tendency. Genu valgum is frequently associated with severely pronated feet in overweight children who begin ambulation at an early age.[4] Pronated feet in children vary from rigid flatfoot to congenital flatfoot (Fig. 8–2) to acquired flatfoot; pronated feet may also be a result of internal tibial torsion. Genu valgum may be secondary to rickets, fractures of the femur, trauma to the epiphyseal plate, paralysis due to lower motor neuron disease, cerebral palsy, or a hip defect, or it may merely be idiopathic. It is most frequently noted between the ages

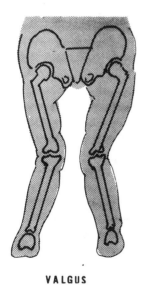 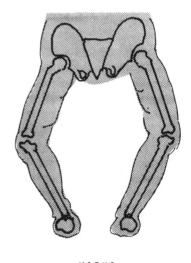

VALGUS   VARUS

Figure 8–1. Genu valgus and genu varus. (*Left*) Genu valgus with the knees close to each other and the ankles separated. (*Right*) Genu varus showing knees separated and ankles together.

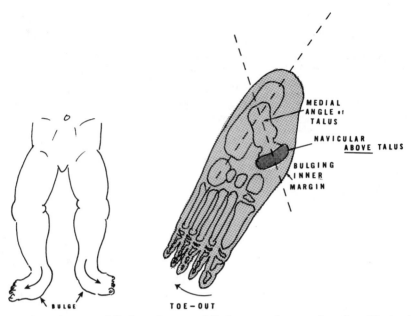

Figure 8–2. Congenital flatfoot. Congenital flatfoot is a calcaneovalgus foot. The heel is in valgus and the talus points medially toward the other foot, forming an angle with the calcaneus. The talus points *downward* rather than forward and the navicular lies on the superior surface of the neck of the talus instead of anterior to the head.

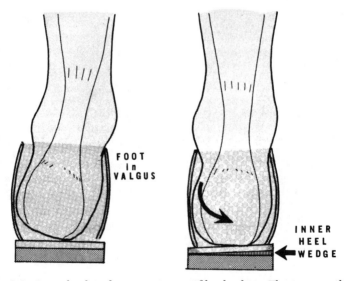

Figure 8–3. Inner heel wedge in treatment of heel valgus. The inner wedge should taper from no elevation at the outer border to $^1/16$ to $^3/16$ in on the inner border. The exact elevation is determined by the height needed to place the calcaneus in a near-vertical position.

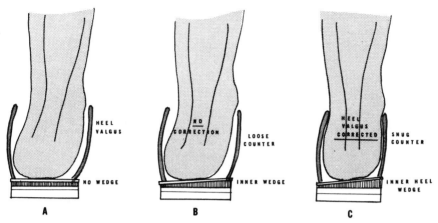

Figure 8–4. The need for a snug heel in correcting heel valgus. (*A*) A valgus heel within a regular shoe. (*B*) An inner wedge in the heel of a loose-fitting shoe does *not* correct the valgus. (*C*) To be effective an inner wedge has to be placed on a shoe counter that "hugs" the heel.

of 2 and 6 and is of major concern to parents when it persists after the age of 6.

Treatment consists of placing an inner wedge of stiff, ⅛-in counter in the snug shoes (Figs. 8–3 and 8–4). The parents should be taught to passively stretch the foot (Fig. 8–5) and encouraged to help the child lose weight.

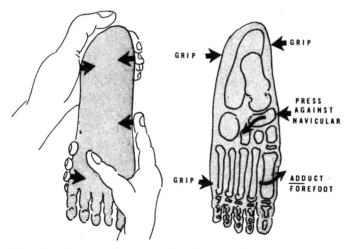

Figure 8–5. Forming an arch in a flatfoot by stretching. Illustration depicts the technique of stretching the right foot. The heel is gripped by the *left* hand holding the calcaneus in a neutral position. The index finger of the *right* hand presses against the navicular bone while the fingers of the *right* hand adduct the forefoot around the fulcrum of the index finger pressing the navicular area. For the left foot the procedure is reversed. In the illustration the right foot is viewed from above.

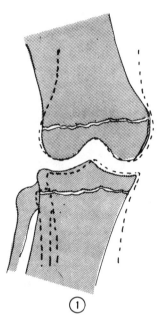

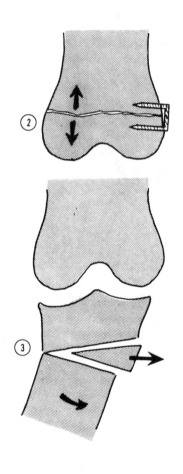

Figure 8–6. Surgical treatment of valgus or varus. (*1*) The knee joint in genu valgus with the open epiphyseal line of the distal femur and proximal tibia. (*2*) Stapling in which the growth on the convex side is stopped, permitting continued growth on the other side (*arrows*). The stapling is left in place until alignment is achieved. (*3*) Osteotomy of the tibia in which a wedge is removed to place the distal portion under the proximal portion, causing the leg to be realigned.

The prognosis depends on the etiological factors, the severity of the valgus, and the inflexibility of the involved tissues. If the ankle malleoli are less than 3 in apart when the child is standing, then conservative treatment or natural development usually produces good results.

In severe genu valgum, surgery may be required. The surgery may consist of stapling the epiphysis or performing an osteotomy (Fig. 8–6). Before stapling, the remaining growth must be calculated. Osteotomy requires that careful measurement be done to correct the valgus (or varus).

GENU VARUM

Genu varum is an abnormality of the alignment of the leg in which the knees are widely separated when the feet are together and the ankle malleoli are in contact. This condition is commonly called bowleg.

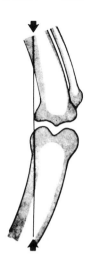

Figure 8–7. X-ray evidence of cortical thickening in valgus. It is on the concave side as a result of the stress of weight bearing.

All normal babies, at birth and during infancy, have some degree of genu varum. The condition frequently persists during the first 3 years of life. Much of the varus is apparent rather than actual and is a result of the normal distribution of thigh fat, the position of the legs caused by the placement of thick diapers, and early weight bearing in chubby children. The apparent condition is aggravated by the coexistence of tibial or femoral torsion.

Physiological bowing (valgus) is symmetrical and involves curving of both the tibia and the femur. X-ray films of this condition usually reveal cortical thickening of the medial (concave) side of the bones (Fig. 8–7). Although most genu varum is physiologically caused, it may be caused by a vitamin D deficiency, renal rickets, osteochondritis (Blount's disease[5]), dyschondroplasia, osteogenesis imperfecta, epiphyseal injury, or neurofibromatosis.

Proper diagnosis is mandatory for proper treatment, but certain principles affect the outcome of any treatment. It is usually desirable to avoid precocious walking, ensure the proper bed position of the newborn, avoid excessive diaper thickness, and institute early and gentle stretching exercises by the parents. Braces are advocated for a moderate to significant abnormality that persists in later childhood (Fig. 8–8).

TIBIAL TORSION

Tibial torsion is not a knee abnormality but is a deviation of the tibia that is "twisted" on its longitudinal axis. This twisting of the tibia in the coronal plane causes the medial malleoli of the ankles to lie in a different plane than the lateral malleoli. If there is internal rotation, the medial malleolus is

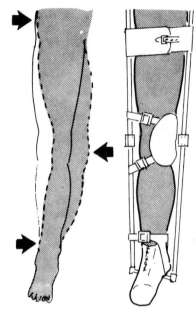

Figure 8–8. Brace treatment of valgus. A long leg brace can be constructed that has three points of pressure (*arrows*) to correct valgus (or varus in reversed manner).

behind the lateral malleolus. This condition exists in the fetus, but at birth the malleoli are on an equal plane. By walking age, 20° of external rotation is considered normal. Khermosh[6] indicated that newborns have an external rotation of 2.2° that gradually externally rotates at an angle of 1.3° per year. Many investigators and clinicians deny the presence of tibial torsion in any direction.

Most tibial torsion is a self-limiting physiological condition that may be a result of internal or external rotation of the hip. Significant internal tibial torsion is associated with bowing, metatarsus varus, or talipes equinovarus (clubfoot) (Fig. 8–9). External rotation is often associated with knock-knee deformities.

Evidence for the presence of the condition is obtained by observing the leg, determining whether the patella is on the inside or outside of the midline (Fig. 8–10), and determining the direction of the foot relative to the midline. The gait must be evaluated for a condition termed "pigeon-toed" (inversion) or a Charlie Chaplin (eversion) type of gait.

If the condition is mild and not of significant cosmetic concern, and if the gait abnormality is acceptable, then no treatment is needed. Otherwise, the parents can perform manipulative exercises of the forefoot. Shoes that correct the inversion or eversion should also be used. Denis-Browne splints (Fig. 8–11) have been in vogue for many years, but their use has been questioned since they apply stress to the knee joints and not to the tibia. In severe gait abnormalities twister braces (Fig. 8–12) have also been advocated, but they are cumbersome, and their efficacy has been questioned.

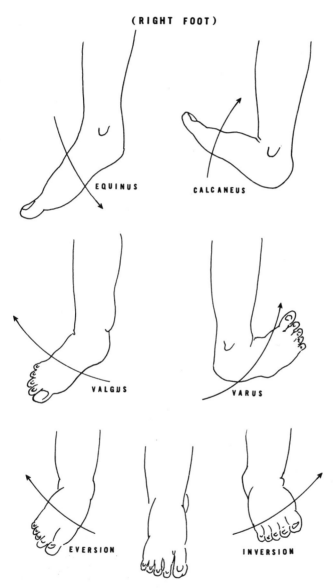

Figure 8–9. Terminology of foot abnormalities or positions.

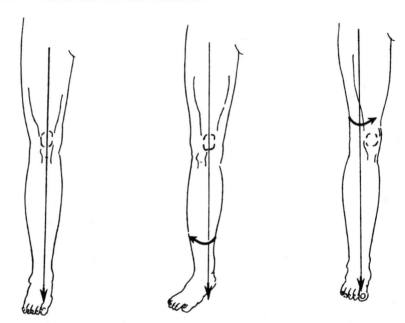

Figure 8–10. Tibial and femoral torsion. The figure to the left shows the "normal" leg in which a plumb line transects the patella and touches the foot between the first and second toes. The middle figure depicts external torsion of the leg with the tibial tubercle being externally placed to the plumb line. The figure on the right depicts internal femoral torsion.

TIBIAL VARUM

Angular deformities can occur in any plane, but the majority are in the coronal plane (valgus or varus) or the sagittal plane (recurvatum). A form of tibial varus that merits separate consideration and causes significant, potentially progressive bowing results from osteochondrosis (osteochondro-

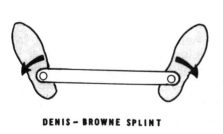

DENIS – BROWNE SPLINT

Figure 8–11. Denis-Browne night splints. The Denis-Browne splint is a pair of shoes for varus or valgus of the foot. The shoes are separated by a specific degree of rotation by bending the bar. The length of the bar is equal to the desired separation of the legs as is the degree of external rotation. The bar places rotatory stress at the knee and may not influence tibial torsion.

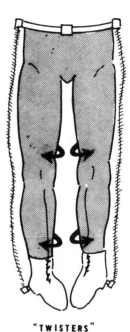

Figure 8–12. Twister braces. Attached to a pelvic band and fixed to the shoe, the twister brace is a set of bilateral spring cables in a housing that tends to rotate the leg externally. The main value of this brace appears to be in the training of an inverted gait toward more external rotation. Its static correction is doubtful.

"TWISTERS"

sis deformans tibiae or Blount's disease). In osteochondrosis deformans tibial there is a disturbance of growth involving the metaphysis epiphyseal cartilage and the osseous center of the epiphysis. Since the pathological condition is located on the medial side of the proximal tibial epiphysis and causes impaired growth, the end result is an abrupt, angular deformity. This condition may be unilateral, but 50 percent of the cases are bilateral (Fig. 8–13).

The criteria of osteochondrosis are:

1. A sharp angular deformity immediately below the proximal tibial epiphysis
2. An irregular epiphyseal cartilage
3. A wedged-shaped osseous portion of the epiphysis
4. A beak projection forming from the medial epiphysis
5. Lax medial ligaments

The onset is insidious. If it is bilateral, the child develops a waddle gait; if it is unilateral, the child develops a limp. Clinically, the leg reveals a sharp angular deformity below the knee. The condition is confirmed by appropriate x-ray findings.

Treatment is expectant with periodic observation. Since this deformity does not progress after the epiphysis is closed, any treatment would be for an

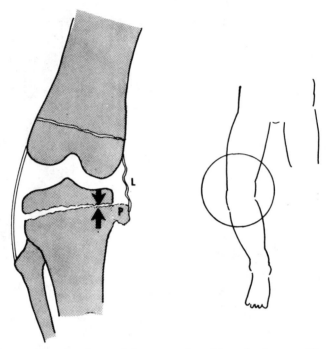

Figure 8–13. Osteochondrosis deformans tibia: Blount's disease. This entity,[5] described by W. Blount, is medial osteochondrosis with sharp angular deformity immediately below the proximal tibial epiphysis, an irregular medial cartilage, the medial metaphysis forming a beaklike projection (P), and lax medial ligaments (L).

associated condition such as severe pronation. Surgical correction of the varum by, for example, osteotomy, must be delayed until epiphyseal closure is evident on x-ray films.

GENU RECURVATUM

Genu recurvatum, a posterior angulation of the knee, has numerous causes, ranging from intrinsic pathological conditions of the knee to secondary factors. The most common cause is a fixed or limited plantar condition of the foot and ankle called equinus. Because of limited dorsiflexion while walking or standing, the knee hyperextends to compensate (see Chap. 9 for details). The excessive plantar flexion may be contractural in origin or result from neurological spasticity. In the resultant hyperextended knee the posterior capsular tissues become elongated and the musculature cannot correct the condition. Flexion contraction may occur after prolonged immobilization during a prolonged illness that requires an inappropriate bed position or postfracture states.

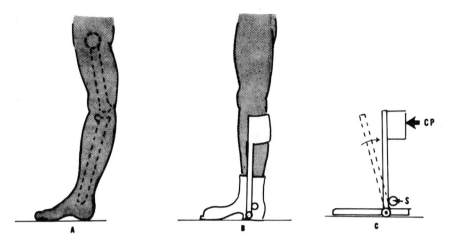

Figure 8–14. Treatment of (*A*) genu recurvatum by a short leg brace. (*B*) The brace has a down-stop at the ankle. By decreasing equinus and thus secondary back knee, it may be effective in preventing recurvatum. (*C*) Mechanical principle of the brace: the stop (*S*); calf pressure (*CP*); and the allowable excursion (*curved arrow*) of the upright bars of the brace on the fixed foot to the floor.

Either the knee or the causative factors (foot-ankle equinus) are treated. The general principles involved are depicted in Figure 8–14. If a frail musculature is responsible for the recurvatum and equinovarus (which result from, for example, peripheral neuropathy, poliomyelitis, and Guillain-Barré syndrome), then the flaccidity must be treated and an appropriate knee brace (Fig. 8–15) should be used. If contracture from prolonged immobiliza-

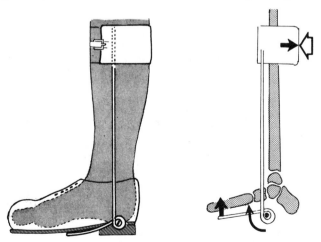

Figure 8–15. Piano wire dorsiflexion brace. When the gastrocnemius has minimal spasticity or in a flaccid drop foot, the resilient piano wire elevates the anterior portion of the foot so it clears the floor during walking.

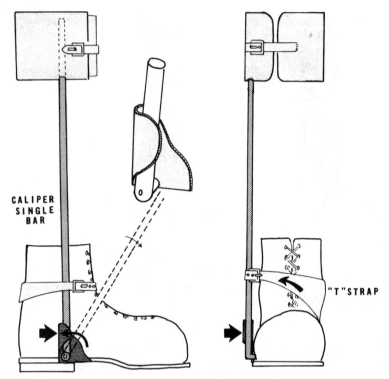

Figure 8–16. Short leg brace with right-angle stop. This short leg brace stops plantar flexion of the foot at a right angle to prevent drop foot or equinus. It may have a single or a double upright bar. The pull of the "T" strap corrects the inversion when it is connected to an inside bar.

tion or a severe neurological spasticity is responsible for the condition, then serial casts may be needed for the offending foot-ankle contracture along with a brace[7–9] for the knee (Fig. 8–16). A tight heel cord that needs stretching and assistance while walking can be treated with an Achilles-tendon-stretching night brace (Fig. 8–17). Local bracing of the knee is effective only during walking but presents problems while sitting (Fig. 8–18).

PAGET'S DISEASE

Paget's disease of the bone is known to have been present in prehistoric times.[10] The histopathology of Paget's disease is characterized by an abundance of osteoclasts and osteoblasts with the bone marrow being invaded by fibrous tissue and numerous blood vessels. Osteoclasts are cells that play an important role in bone resorption. In the early phase of the disease there is an increase in osteoclastic activity with bone resorption, and

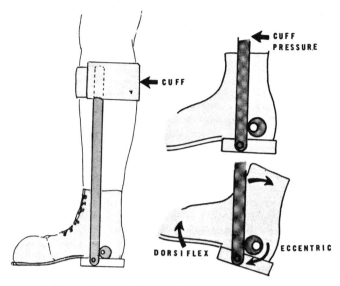

Figure 8–17. Achilles tendon-stretching night brace. The eccentric ankle joint forces the bar to varying degrees, altering the ankle dorsiflexion. The cuff affords counter pressure. In the right lower picture the rotation of the eccentric joint has forced the foot into dorsiflexion.

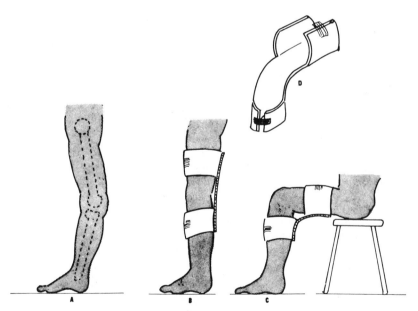

Figure 8–18. Back heel brace for genu recurvatum. (*A*) The usual back knee stance, regardless of the etiologic factors. Brace is designed to control recurvatum while standing (*B*) and to permit sitting (*C*). (*D*) The brace is a dynamic splint made of orthoplast with 25° flexion molded into splint. (Adapted from Andersen, CB: Dynamic knee splint to prevent hyperextension. Phys Ther 52:944, 1972.)

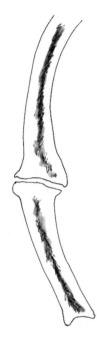

Figure 8–19. Radiological aspect of Paget's disease of the lower extremity. The femur and tibia are curved, and the cortex of the bone is thickened and hypercalcified. The marrow is trabecular in appearance with hypervascularization. The knee has undergone severe degenerative changes.

in the later phase compensatory bone formation from excessive osteoblastic activity results in a mosaic pattern. The final, "burned out" phase is characterized by a dense mosaic bone with little or no cellular activity.

Clinically the patient with Paget's disease presents with progressive deformity of the long bones. Pain may be present, but a large number of patients with Paget's disease have no pain. Pain is believed to result from the stretching of the periosteum over the pagetoid bone, which in turn may stimulate somatic sensory nerve endings. In advanced stages there may be a typical bowing of a leg due to involvement of the tibia or femur (Fig. 8–19).

The knee in Paget's disease resembles that seen in severe degenerative arthritis, especially if the pagetoid changes occur in the bone adjacent to the joint. The patella may also undergo pagetoid changes that cause chondropatellar arthritic pain and impairment.

Although the treatment of Paget's disease remains unpredictable and is often disappointing, a major advance in its treatment has been the introduction of calcitonin.[10] Calcitonin essentially inhibits bone resorption, increases urinary excretion of sodium, calcium, phosphorus, and uric acid, which may significantly influence bone changes as noted on x-ray films, and affords relief of bone pain. The dosage of calcitonin depends on the commercial source of the hormone and must be monitored carefully by an internist, oncologist, or endocrinologist who has experience using the drug.

Correction of bone deformity presents significant problems since the disease occurs in elderly people who also present problems of bleeding from the hypervascular bone that is characteristic of Paget's disease and have a tendency for delayed healing or nonunion. In the tibia and femur, osteotomy has been successful in realigning the bones of the leg and relieving the knee pain. Total hip replacement has also been very effective and may relieve pressure on the knee. There are reports that sarcoma results from operated and/or manipulated Paget's bones, but this has been refuted.[11]

REFERENCES

1. Stelling, FH: General affections of the skeletal system. Pediatr Clin North Amer 14:3559, 1967.
2. Rubin, P: Dynamic Classification of Bone Dysplasia. Yearbook Medical Publishers, Chicago, 1964.
3. Thomas, CL (ed): Taber's Cyclopedic Medical Dictionary, ed 15. FA Davis, Philadelphia, 1985.
4. Cailliet, R: The foot in childhood. In Cailliet, R (ed): Foot and Ankle Pain, FA Davis, Philadelphia, 1968, p 57.
5. Blount, WP: Tibia vara. J Bone Joint Surg 19:1, 1937.
6. Khermosh, O, Lior, G, and Weisman, SL: Tibial torsion in children. Clin Orthop 79:25, 1971.
7. Smith, EM and Juvinall, RR: Mechanics of bracing. In Licht, S (ed): Orthotics Etcetera. Waverly Press, Baltimore, 1966.
8. Perry, J: Orthopedic management of the lower extremity in the hemiplegic patient. J Amer Phys Therap 46:345, 1966.
9. Stamp, W: Bracing in cerebral palsy. J Bone Joint Surg 44A:1457, 1962.
10. Singer, FR: Paget's Disease of Bone. Plenum Medical Book Company, New York, 1977.
11. Barry, HC: Paget's Disease of Bone. Williams & Wilkins, Baltimore, 1969.

CHAPTER 9

The Knee in Gait:
Normal and Abnormal

The functional knee in stance and gait in childhood and adulthood must be understood before specifics of the abnormal gait and stance can be evaluated and remedied. All aspects of the trunk and lower extremities, especially the knee, are involved in the synchronous coordinated gait. Factors to be considered are neuromuscular coordination, quadriceps competency, hamstring muscle group involvement, articular range adequacy, structural tissue normalcy within the knee, proprioceptive adequacy, training compliance, and involvement of the foot and hip joints. All of these must be considered when evaluating the knee function in gait and stance.

NORMAL GAIT

There are determinants[1] in the normal gait that attempt to minimize vertical body displacement to decrease energy expenditure. The trunk shifts from side to side with simultaneous axial and sagittal rotation, undergoing approximately 2 cm of displacement. The body weight supported at the sacrum-pelvis, consisting of the trunk, head, and the upper extremities, is 50 percent of the total body weight. During the swing phase of gait, the swinging leg adds another 15 percent of body weight. At the one-leg stance phase during gait, 85 percent of the total body weight must be balanced on that one leg. The determinants are quite economically effective at limiting the amount of weight that is lifted at every phase of gait.

Forward gait motion is initiated by shifting the trunk's center of gravity forward. The leg swings forward to prevent a fall or loss of balance. This is considered the *swing phase*. The hip flexes approximately 20° with the knee

262

slightly flexed to assist the foot and toe in clearing the floor. When the leg has completed the swing phase, the body mass is forward and the swing leg undergoes a *heel strike* (Fig. 9–1). The foot is dorsiflexed and the knee is fully extended. Impact to the body is dampened by the knee, which is slightly flexed (15°), and by the heel pad. This is the beginning of the *stance phase*. The forward leg becomes weight bearing and the knee gradually fully extends. This knee extension occurs because the posterior leg tissues, the gastrocnemius-soleus muscle complex, apply posterior "pull" on the upper aspect of the lower leg. It is virtually a passive knee extension as the body passes over the center of gravity.

At midstance, the body is directly over the center of gravity and the foot is flat on the floor with no significant ankle plantar or dorsiflexion. The foot has been in the inverted (supinated) position (Fig. 9–2) during the entire swing phase and at heel strike, but as the foot becomes weight bearing, it pronates to full pronation. The knee at midstance (Fig. 9–3) is fully extended (with the quadriceps not contracted). The knee remains extended until there is resumption of the swing phase in the next step in the gait.[2,3]

There is rotation of the pelvis, femur, and tibia during these gait phases. The pelvis, femur, and tibia rotate 8°, 8°, and 9°, respectively, for a total of 25°. From the beginning of the onset of the swing phase, all the rotation is in an internal direction until midphase, when all the rotation is outward until the push off. During this rotation the femur and the tibia are disproportionally rotated,[4] indicating that there is rotation at the knee of the tibia on the femoral condyles.

The muscular action on the knee in normal gait is as follows. At the initiation of the swing, the short head of the biceps (hamstring group), the gracilis, and the sartorius contract in an attempt to decelerate the swing or at least moderate its force. The last-mentioned two muscles essentially extend the leg at the knee and direct its path forward. The quadriceps undergoes contraction to assist in hip flexion. As heel strike approaches, the quadriceps contracts maximally to absorb the shock and then relaxes to decelerate knee flexion (15°), which decreases the body's elevation during midstance (Fig. 9–4).

The rectus femoris becomes active again during the midstance phase,[2] when there is a slight flexion, and remains active when the hip flexes (end of the stance phase) to initiate the next swing phase.

The hamstring group of muscles has a peak of contraction (Fig. 9–5) during the swing phase to decelerate the leg and peaks again when the foot is firmly planted on the ground to prevent the knee (and hip) from buckling (i.e., further flexion). The hamstrings are essentially decelerators as well as a possible source of kinesthetic proprioception. It is apparent from their contribution to gait that these muscles require adequate elongation.

The muscular activities of the ankle, hip, and pelvis during gait will not be discussed here except as they relate to knee activities. At heel strike the hip extensors bring the body forward above the weight-bearing leg (Fig.

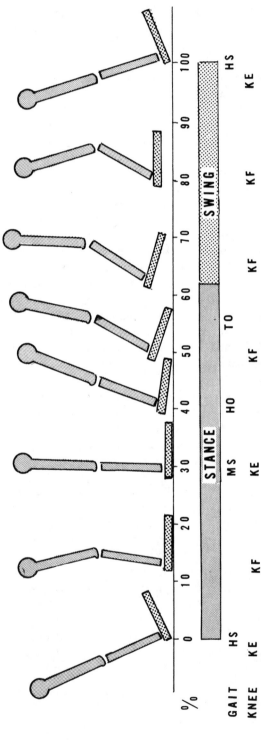

Figure 9–1. Gait cycle. The percentage (%) denotes the increments of a full gait cycle—in this figure the right leg in one cycle. HS is heel strike, beginning the stance phase (0%). At heel strike, the knee is extended (KE). As the body passes over the weight-bearing leg, the knee flexes slightly (KF) to absorb shock. At midstance (MS 30%), the knee is fully extended (KE). At heel-off (HO 40%), the knee begins to flex slightly (KF 50%) and remains flexed through toe-off (TO 62%), when the swing phase begins. The knee remains flexed throughout swing phase until preheel strike, when the knee re-extends (KE 100%).

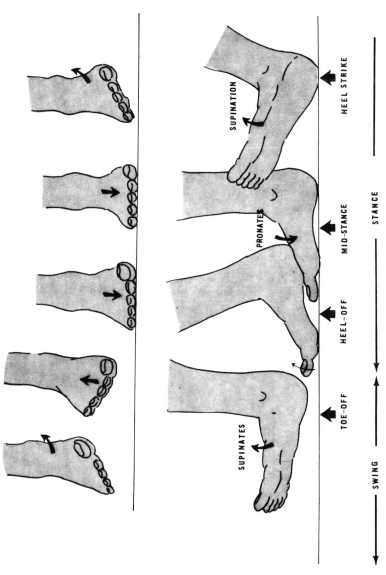

Figure 9–2. Foot during stance phase. The heel strike to flatfoot occurs at 7 percent of the gait cycle through 12 percent; at 35 percent, the heel leaves the floor (heel-off). Toe-off starts the swing phase of that leg and begins at 60 percent of the full gait cycle.

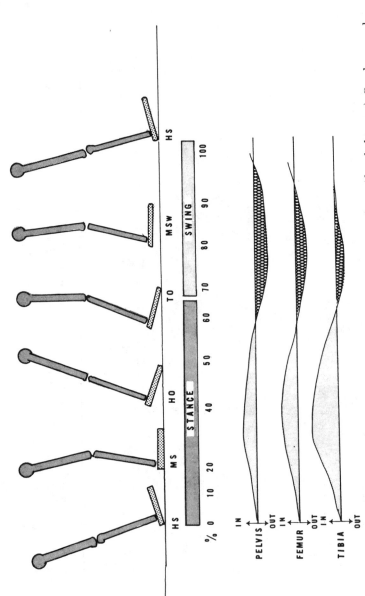

Figure 9–3. Knee in gait. The gait is shown depicting the stance and swing phases (detailed in text). One leg spends 60 percent of gait in stance (weight bearing) from heel strike (HS) through midstance (MS), heel-off (HO), and, ultimately, toe-off (TO). The swing phase then begins through midswing phase (MSW) to end at heel strike (HS). The knee bends 20° at MS, again at TO through MSW; otherwise it is extended. During gait, the pelvis, femur, and tibia, each slightly independent, undergo internal rotation (IN) during the stance phase as the body passes over the weight-bearing leg. Just before the beginning of the swing phase (50%) and through the swing phase, the pelvis, femur, and tibia rotate externally (OUT), with the tibia rotating more than the femur. Rotatory torque occurs at the knee.

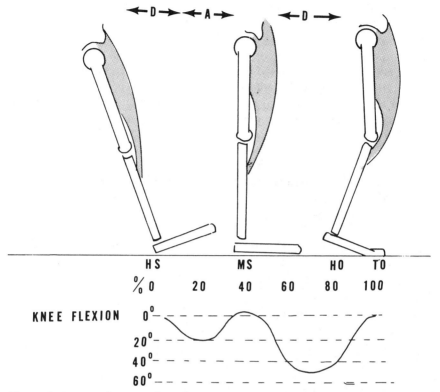

Figure 9–4. Knee flexion and quadriceps action in gait. At heel strike (HS) at the beginning of the stance phase (0%), the quadriceps are contracted; this decelerates (D) as the knee flexes. At midstance (MS 40%), the quadriceps has actively extended the knee (A). As the stance phase progresses, the knee again flexes, but more (to 60°), and again the quadriceps decelerates flexion. After toe-off (TO 100%), the leg is in swing phase and quadriceps actively extends the knee and swings the leg forward. The stickman figures here are not directly above the graphs or the numerals.

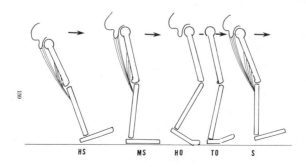

Figure 9–5. Action of hamstrings in gait. The hamstrings decelerate the leg at the termination of the swing phase (S) prior to heel strike (HS). During the stance phase at midpoint (MP), the hamstrings presumably assist in hip extension.

9–6). Good hip extensors and proprioceptive sensation extend the hip and pull the thigh posteriorly over the fixed foot and ankle. The extended knee "locks" on its soft tissue (capsule and ligaments), decreasing the need for strong quadriceps contraction.

The lower leg influences the knee during gait in that the gastrocnemius-soleus muscles contract to pull the lower leg posteriorly over the fixed foot during the stance phase (Fig. 9–7). The gastrocnemius-soleus muscles also become active in the push-off phase of gait.

ABNORMAL GAIT: NEUROLOGICAL AND ORTHOPEDIC

Pathological gait is a result of:

1. A structural abnormality in which there is a change in the length or shape of the bones of the lower extremity
2. A pathological change of the soft tissue of the lower extremity, primarily of the articular structures
3. A neuromuscular disorder in which the control of the gait is abnormal

Structural Changes

Inequality in the length of the legs will cause gait abnormality. The pelvis on the short side drops, causing the opposite leg to compensate. The unaffected (longer) leg undergoes an increase in knee, hip, and ankle flexion during the swing phase, and there is a tendency for the short leg to compensate by initiating toe walking with slight knee hyperextension.

Soft Tissue Pathology

An inflammatory disease of joints, particularly of the knee, impairs the gait. There is a reduction in gait velocity, knee flexion, and full extension: all are influenced by a diminution of impact on the ground at the heel strike and midstance phases.

In a contracted joint, such as the hip joint with varying degrees of ankylosis, the knee (and the low back) compensates by placing added stress on the ipsilateral knee and the contralateral hip during gait. If the knee is contracted, the limb is shortened in its length and a short-leg limp results. This is more apparent at faster walking speeds and with a contracture of 30°. If the knee is contracted in extension, it presents a gait that is similar to the

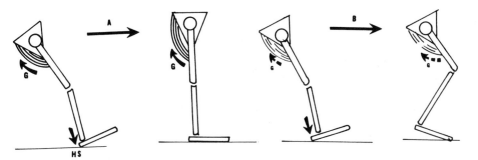

Figure 9–6. Gait analysis. (*A*) Normal gait with heel strike (HS), the knee slightly flexed to dampen the impact. The hip extensors (G) extend the hip and pull the pelvis over the weight-bearing leg at the stance phase. (*B*) Gait with weak gluteal (hip) extensors (G) that fail to extend the hip, and thus at stance phase the knee is still flexed as the pelvis passes over the fixed foot. (*Right*) The foot is in equinus stance and is not related to the hip weakness.

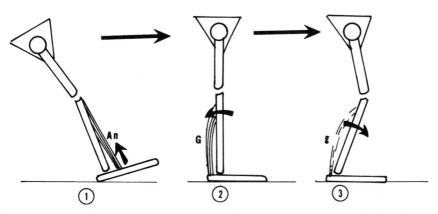

Figure 9–7. Effect of weak soleus gait on the knee. (*1*) The anticus (ankle dorsiflexor) (An) at heel strike prevents foot slap. (*2*) As the pelvis passes over the fixed foot during the stance phase the gastrocnemius-soleus muscle (G) prevents excessive ankle dorsiflexion and decelerates the leg as it passes over the fixed foot. This action simultaneously prevents the knee from flexing in stance. (*3*) With a weak soleus (g) excessive ankle dorsiflexion occurs and the knee flexes unless strong quadriceps or strong hip extensors or both intervene.

one seen when one leg is longer and is thus compensated by circumduction and hip hike during the swing-through phase. During the stance phase, the pelvis and center of gravity rise more since knee and hip flexion does not happen at midstance. Also the heel strike is more forceful since there is no knee flexion to dampen the impact.

Equinus, from spasticity, Achilles tendon contracture, or ankle foot arthrodesis, causes the leg to be too long in all phases of gait. Thus, excessive knee and hip flexion and a potential back knee (recurvatum) during the stance phase are required. Joint instability from excessive laxity or proprioceptive deficiency results in excessive joint motion during weight bearing and in *buckling* during the stance phase.

Painful weight bearing causes an antalgic gait, that is, a gait that attempts to avoid the pain. Short steps are taken to minimize the pain and all aspects of the gait may be exaggerated in this attempt. The painful knee is usually held in a slightly flexed position with avoidance of full extension.

Neuromuscular Defects

Paresis causing loss of muscular contracture during gait impairs the gait. Weakness of the gastrocnemius-soleus complex adversely affects the knee during gait. Weakness or paralysis of this muscle group can result from central nervous system diseases such as poliomyelitis, Guillin-Barré syndrome, diabetic neuropathy, spinal cord injury, or residual nerve root damage from a cord tumor or ruptured disc. The neurological examination together with the history will identify the disease that is causing the paresis. Besides problems with gait, the patient is unable to stand on his or her toes, and the ankle jerk is absent.

The knee does not fully extend, that is, it remains slightly flexed, placing excessive demands on the quadriceps during standing and walking. Adequate strength of the hip and ankle musculature can compensate for 15° of knee flexion from a capsular contracture or bone abnormality. The quadriceps can be paretic from nerve root (femoral) involvement that results from a systemic disease such as rheumatoid arthritis, diabetes, or poliomyelitis. Regardless of whether the cause is a flexion contraction or a paretic knee extension, the flexed knee and hip throughout the gait shift the center of gravity forward (Fig. 9–8). A sustained flexed knee posture or stance resulting from impaired knee extension causes excessive strain on the extensor mechanisms of the remaining knee and permits buckling at stance phase.

An equinus of the foot and ankle caused by paresis of the dorsiflexors or a contracted Achilles tendon or gastrocnemius-soleus muscle group results in

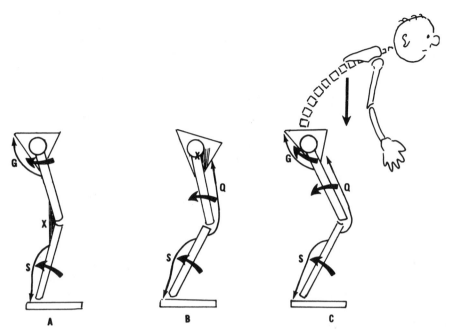

Figure 9–8. Pathologic stance phase of gait. (*A*) Flexed knee stance caused by contracture (X) of the knee. Erect stance is possible with strong hip extensors (G, gluteals) and strong plantar flexors (S, soleus). (*B*) Flexed stance as a result of hip flexion contracture (X) overcome by strong quadriceps (Q) and strong soleus (S). The former extends the knee and the latter pulls the leg back over the fixed foot. (*C*) Flexed stance resulting from bent-over posture with most of the body weight (60 to 65 percent) placed ahead of the center of gravity. All the extensors are needed to maintain an erect stance.

an abnormal gait since dorsiflexion during the swing phase is prevented and the foot cannot clear the floor. A persistent equinus results in a back knee (recurvatum) during the stance phase and a flexed knee at the end of the stance phase (Fig. 9–9).

Paresis of the ankle dorsiflexors may result from a systemic neurological disease such as amyotrophic lateral sclerosis, poliomyelitis, Guillain-Barré syndrome, or peripheral neuropathy. A careful neurological examination will indicate the diagnosis and an electromyographic examination will confirm the affected nerve roots.[5,6]

A patient with a flaccid paralysis but who retains normal proprioception may be able to compensate for the deficit. However, if this is not happening, then a brace may be needed to compensate for the sensory and motor deficit.

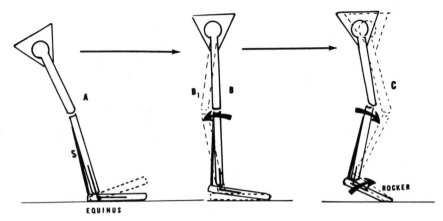

Figure 9–9. Equinus gait: contracted or spastic soleus. (A) There is no heel strike because the foot is in equinus during the swing phase. (B) Normally extended knee. As the pelvis passes over the fixed foot, the shortened soleus extends the knee mechanically. If the equinus is excessive (B_1), back knee (hyperextension) can occur (*broken line*). (C) In a marked equinus during the last part of the stance phase, the foot can rock over the weight-bearing toes and throw the pelvis ahead of the center of gravity. This imposes marked stress upon the quadriceps or permits falling if the quadriceps is inadequate.

THE KNEE IN A SPASTIC GAIT

The completed stroke[7] initially involves a flaccid lower extremity[8] that gradually progresses into a spastic then synergistic phase. The process of extension includes extension and internal rotation of the hip, extension of the knee, and the equinovarus position of the foot and ankle. The hemiparetic spastic gait is slow and poorly coordinated. Because of an extensor spastic leg, the leg cannot flex and thus must circumduct to advance. The straight knee causes an excessive rise of the pelvis and thus an increased elevation in the center of gravity. There is a shortened heel strike phase with the forefoot striking before the heel. This aspect of gait can be partially controlled by an appropriate brace.[9,10]

CONCLUSION

Careful evaluation of the function and malfunction of the knee requires:

1. A neurological examination for motor paresis or hyperreflexia with or without proprioceptive loss

2. An orthopedic evaluation for contracture, malalignment, or excessive laxity

3. A careful evaluation of stance and gait[11]

4. Appropriate tests to complement the neurological examination

The medical, neurological, or orthopedic elements responsible for the abnormal gait should be treated first. Then the patient should be introduced to and instructed in appropriate rehabilitation techniques aimed at improving the gait. In the young patient with spastic paralysis, such as with cerebral palsy, surgical interventions aim at decreasing the deforming conditions that cause a scissor gait (Fig. 9–10). Release of the deforming spastic muscles at their sites of attachment or eliminating their innervation (with nerve blocks and disrupters) may be needed to prevent long-term deformity from the continuing muscular imbalance. The posture resulting from a severe spastic condition (such as cerebral palsy) may be ameliorated by Eggers' procedure (Fig. 9–11).[14]

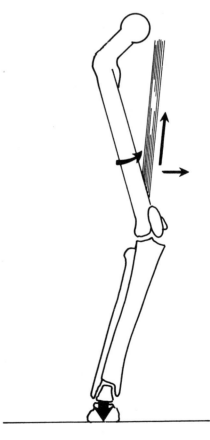

Figure 9–10. Internal femoral torsion from adductor mechanism. When the foot is fixed to the floor (*arrow*) and the knee and hip flexed in the crouch position of cerebral palsy, the adductors that act on the leg cause valgus at the knee and internally rotate the femur. If this occurs bilaterally, the classic scissor gait results.

"CROUCH"

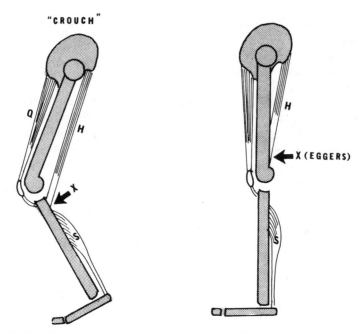

Figure 9–11. Crouch position in spastic cerebral palsy: Eggers' procedure. (*Left*) Crouch posture caused by spastic hamstrings (H) flexing the knee. There is a simultaneous hip flexion and foot equinus. (*Right*) By transplanting the hamstring insertions from the tibia to the posterior femur, knee flexion is eliminated. The hips thus extend more, and the equinus is improved or is corrected.

REFERENCES

1. Saunders, JB deCM, Inman, VT, and Eberhart, HD: Major determinants in normal and pathological gait. J Bone Joint Surg 35A:543, 1953.
2. Lehmann, JF and DeLateur, BJ: Gait analysis: Diagnosis and management. In Kottke, FJ and Lehmann, JF (eds): Krusen's Handbook of Physical Medicine and Rehabilitation, ed 4. WB Saunders, Philadelphia, 1990, p 108.
3. Inman, VT, Ralston, HJ, and Todd, F: Human Walking. Williams & Wilkins, Baltimore, 1981.
4. Levens, AS, Inman, VT, and Blosser, JA: Transverse rotation of the segments of the lower extremity in locomotion. J Bone Joint Surg 30A:859, 1948.
5. Basmajian, JV: Muscles Alive: Their Function Revealed by Electromyography. Williams & Wilkins, Baltimore, 1962.
6. Liberson, WT: Biomechanics of gait: A method of study. Arch Phys Med Rehab 48:37, 1965.
7. Davies, PM: Steps to Follow: Guide to the Treatment of Adult Hemiplegia. Springer-Verlag, New York, 1985.
8. Cailliet, R: The Shoulder in Hemiplegia. FA Davis, Philadelphia, 1980.
9. Perry, J: Bracing of the knee. J Canadian Phys Therap Assoc 24:298, 1972.
10. Cailliet, R: Bracing for Spasticity. In Licht, S (ed): Orthotics Etcetera. Waverly Press, Baltimore, 1966.

11. Schenker, AW: Pathological implications of abnormal stance and gait. Occup Therap Rehab 28:131, 1949.
12. Bobath, K and Bobath, BA: A treatment of cerebral palsy. Brit J Phys Med 15:105, 1952.
13. Knott, M and Voss, DE: Proprioceptive Neuromuscular Facilitation. Harper & Row, New York, 1968.
14. Eggers, GWN and Evans, EB: Surgery in cerebral palsy: AAOS instructional course lecture. J Bone Joint Surg 45A:1275, 1963.

Index

An "*f*" following a page number indicates a figure.
A "*t*" following a page number indicates a table.